AED/CPR/First Aid Training Manual

A Rescuer's Complete Guide to Emergency Response

||| D1684994

EMS Safety Services

Prepare • Practice • Perform

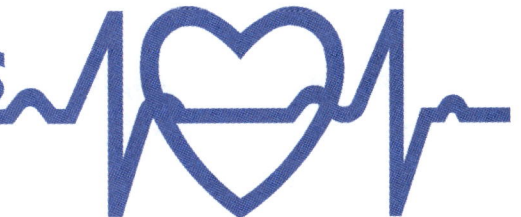

EMS Safety Services, Inc.
1046 Calle Recodo, Suite K
San Clemente, CA 92673
800.215.9555
www.emssafety.com

AED/CPR/First Aid Training Manual
A Rescuer's Complete Guide to Emergency Response

Copyright © 2007 EMS Safety Services, Inc.

ISBN: 978-0-9796966-1-9

EMS Safety Services, Inc.
1046 Calle Recodo, Suite K
San Clemente, CA 92673
800.215.9555 Fax 949.388.2776
www.emssafety.com

The emergency care procedures described in this manual are based on guidelines from the 2005 International Conference on CPR and ECC Science with Treatment Recommendations hosted by the American Heart Association, and the most current accepted standards and information available at the time of publishing. EMS Safety Services does not guarantee or assume responsibility for the completeness, correctness or sufficiency of the information or standards. It is the reader's responsibility to stay informed of changes in recommendations or information on emergency care procedures.

CPR/First Aid training references are available upon request from EMS Safety Services.

CPR/First Aid training materials meet OSHA compliance standards.

Cover photographs by Andrew Baerst

Printed in the United States of America

Introduction

Timely and appropriate bystander care followed by a quick response from professional rescuers gives victims of injury or sudden illness their best chance of survival. Our main objective is to teach basic first aid/CPR/AED skills that can sustain or save a life while professional emergency help is on the way. The goal of our training is to make the home and work environment safer by preventing illness and injury as well as quickly recognizing and responding to emergencies. The content of this book is not meant as a substitute for professional medical advice or treatment.

EMS Safety Services provides basic First Aid, CPR and AED training programs designed by professional emergency care providers. In order to be taught to professional rescuers or health care providers, additional training units are required. The instructor must ensure that the curriculum has been approved for the professional rescuer or health care provider prior to the class. Contact EMS Safety Services headquarters for verification.

This workbook is for you, the student, to keep and use as a reference. Feel free to make notations in the student workbook during the class. To comment on the course, **visit www.emssafety.com to download a course evaluation form**, or call (800) 215-9555.

Thanks for choosing EMS Safety Services, Inc. Enjoy your course.

EMERGENCY ACTION CARD

BASIC RESCUER

CALL 911 FOR MEDICAL EMERGENCIES:

- Difficulty breathing
- Chest pain or discomfort for 5 minutes
- Sudden weakness, slurred speech, severe headache
- Altered mental status, unresponsive
- Severe injury or illness
- Severe bleeding
- Pregnancy emergency
- Critical burn
- Suspected poisoning
- Electrical shock
- Seizure

RECOVERY POSITION

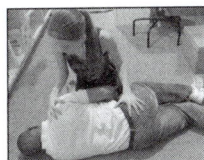

- For unresponsive breathing victims
- Position arm out to side.
- Grasp hip and shoulder.
- Log roll victim to the side.
- Monitor breathing.

BLEEDING CONTROL

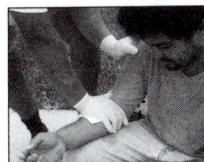

- PPE
- Apply firm, direct pressure.
- Add dressings; do not remove.
- Treat for shock (elevate legs, maintain body temperature).

CPR

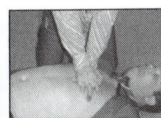

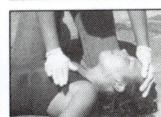

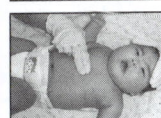

- Establish Response: Tap & Shout
- Call 911 & get AED; send bystander
- A - Open Airway: Head tilt/chin lift
- B - Check Breathing: 5-10 seconds
- Give 2 Breaths
- If breathing, use recovery position
- C - Begin Chest Compressions
- 30 Compressions, 2 Breaths
- Continue Cycles of 30:2
- D - Use AED when arrives
- S - If breathing, assess for Severe bleeding and Shock

CPR TECHNIQUES BY AGE

	Adult	Child	Infant
Age	8+ years	1-8 years	0-1 year
2 Breaths	1 second, Into mouth		1 second, Mouth & Nose
Rate	Compressions at 100/minute		
Technique	2 hands	1-2 hands	2 fingers
Depth	$1^1/_2$ – 2 in.	$1/_3$ to $1/_2$ depth of chest	
Cycles	30:2		
AED	ASAP	After 2 min.	No recommendation

ADULT/CHILD CHOKING

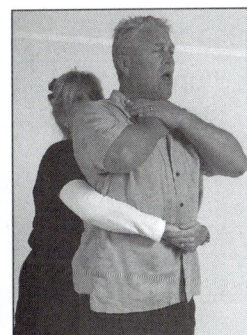

- If victim can speak, encourage cough.

- If unable to speak:
  - Stand behind the victim.
  - Place fist just above navel.
  - Grasp fist with other hand.
  - Abdominal thrusts until relieved.
  - CPR if unresponsive; look for object before breaths.

INFANT CHOKING

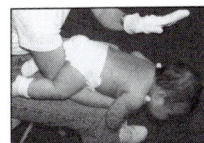

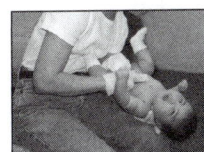

- If victim can cry, do not interfere.

- If unable to cry:
  - Turn face down.
  - Support on thigh.
  - Give 5 sharp back blows.
  - Turn face up.
  - Give 5 chest thrusts.
  - Continuous back blows and chest thrusts.
  - Use CPR if unresponsive.

HEART ATTACK

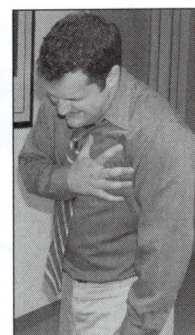

- Assess for symptoms:
  - Chest pain, discomfort
  - Radiating discomfort
  - Shortness of breath
  - Sweating, nausea
  - Dizziness
- Position of comfort.
- Call 911 if symptoms last for 5 minutes.
- Calm and reassure.
- Lay down if dizzy or faint.
- ABCD'S if unresponsive.

STROKE

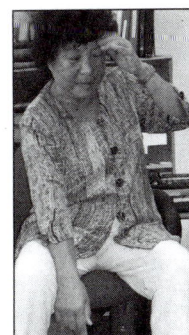

- Sudden onset of symptoms:
  - Headache
  - Facial droop
  - Confusion
  - Slurred speech
  - Weakness/numbness on one side of the body
- Position of comfort.
- Call 911.
- Calm and reassure.
- Recovery position if needed.
- ABCD'S if unresponsive.

EMERGENCY ASSESSMENT FORM

SCENE SIZE-UP

☐ Scene Safety   # of Victims _____

☐ Call 911   ☐ PPE   ☐ Consent   ☐ ABCD 'S

☐ Injury   ☐ Illness

☐ Unknown (treat as Injury)

☐ Hazards (traffic, chemicals, fire, blood)

DESCRIPTION OF INCIDENT

Date _____

Location _____

Description _____

_____

_____

_____

_____

PAIN ASSESSMENT

Chief Complaint _____

_____

Provoke _____

Quality _____

Region/Radiate _____

Severity _____

Time _____

HEAD-TO-TOE ASSESSMENT

If neck pain, stop - stablize head & neck together.

Deformity, Open Wounds, Tenderness, Swelling

1. Neck: D O T S	5. Abdomen: D O T S
2. Head: D O T S	6. Pelvis: D O T S
3. Ears: D O T S	7. Back: D O T S
4. Chest: D O T S	8. Extrem.: D O T S

PATIENT ASSESSMENT   (reassess every 5 minutes)

Time	ABCD'S Intact	Skin Temp warm, cool	Color flushed, pale, bluish	Moisture dry, sweaty	Response alert/altered/unresponsive

PATIENT INFORMATION

Name _____

☐ M ☐ F   Age ____   Tel # _____

Address _____

Contact Person _____

Relationship _____

Tel #_____

MEDICAL HISTORY

Symptoms _____

Allergies _____

Medications _____

Past History _____

Last Oral Intake _____

Events Prior _____

EMS Safety Services, Inc.   **1-800-215-9555**   **www.emssafety.com**

GENERAL INFORMATION

CPR

FIRST AID ASSESSMENT

INJURIES

MEDICAL EMERGENCIES

ENVIRONMENTAL EMERGENCIES

Giving care in an emergency can have a physical, mental and emotional impact on the rescuer. The amount of stress will vary depending on the seriousness of the incident and each rescuer's unique response to it.

SIGNS AND SYMPTOMS:
PHYSICAL RESPONSE

- Rapid breathing or heart rate
- Trembling
- Sweating
- Nausea, diarrhea
- Headache, muscle ache
- Fatigue
- Difficulty sleeping
- Increased or decreased appetite

MENTAL RESPONSE

- Cannot stop thinking about the event
- Confusion, difficulty concentrating
- Nightmares

EMOTIONAL RESPONSE

- Anxiety, worry, guilt, fear, anger
- Depression, crying
- Restlessness
- Change in behavior or interactions with people

A rescuer's response to an incident is usually temporary, lasting just a few days. If the rescuer is unable to cope with the stress produced by the incident, the effects may last for weeks or even months. It can affect his or her health, family life, and work performance.

TIPS FOR STRESS MANAGEMENT:

- Eat properly.
- Avoid alcohol, drugs and caffeine.
- Exercise, and get enough rest.
- Talk about your feelings.
- Don't judge yourself for your actions.
- Obtain professional help if needed.

HEALTH & SAFETY ONLINE RESOURCES

MedlinePlus, U.S. National Library of Medicine, NIH – www.medlineplus.gov

American Association of Poison Control Centers 1.800.222.1222 – www.aapcc.org

Centers for Disease Control and Prevention – www.cdc.gov

American Lung Association Freedom from Smoking® Online – www.lungusa.org

Occupational Safety & Health Administration – www.osha.gov

Substance Abuse & Mental Health Services Administration – www.findtreatment.samhsa.gov

National Highway Traffic Safety Administration – www.nhtsa.dot.gov

U.S. Department of Health and Human Services – www.healthfinder.gov

Heart disease is the leading cause of death among adults in the United States. In many cases, the end result of heart disease is **sudden cardiac arrest (SCA)**. This year over 1.2 million Americans will suffer a heart attack; over 500,000 of these will result in death. Most heart attack-related fatalities occur prior to reaching the hospital or in the emergency department.

The number one enemy during SCA is time. There are four critical interventions to increase a victim's chance of survival. The less time taken between each critical step, the better the odds of survival.

EARLY ACCESS TO CARE (EMS SYSTEM)

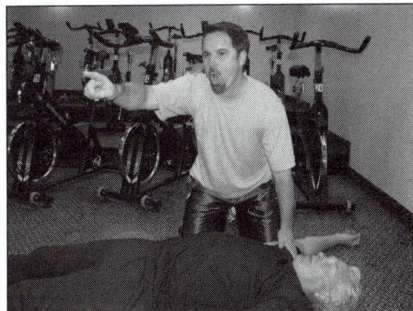

Dialing your local emergency response number, which is 911 in most regions, activates the **Emergency Medical Services system (EMS)**. A dispatcher will send the appropriate emergency personnel to the scene. Always hang up last.

My emergency number is: _____

EARLY CPR

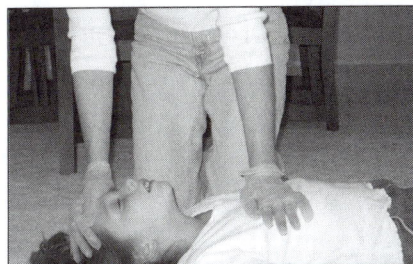

CPR can add a few minutes to the time available for successful defibrillation. For the best chance of survival:

- Start CPR immediately after cardiac arrest.
- Perform chest compressions correctly and with minimal interruptions.

EARLY DEFIBRILLATION

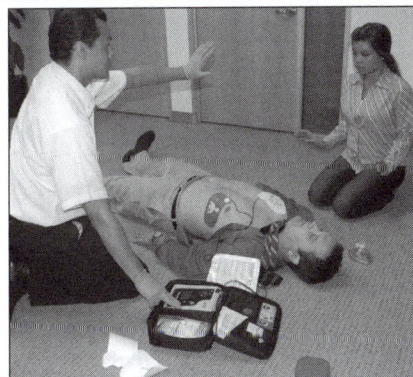

Early defibrillation is the most critical step in increasing the chances of surviving SCA. Defibrillation is most effective when combined with high quality CPR. With each minute that passes without CPR and a shock from a defibrillator, there is a 10% decreased chance of survival.

EARLY ADVANCED CARE

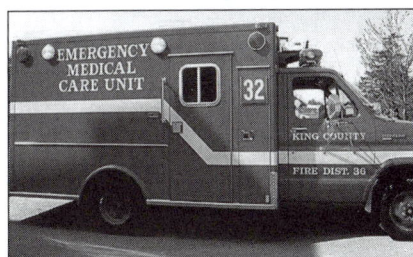

Advanced Life Support, such as advanced airway management and drug therapy, will be provided by specially trained medical professionals on the scene and en route to the hospital.

Decide to Respond:

- Regardless of age, gender, race, ethnicity, or socioeconomic status.
- Even if others are present, or you are uneasy. If unsure of what to do, call 911.

Duty to Act: The responder has a legal obligation to act, according to statute or job description (e.g. professional rescuer, licensed health care provider, public safety first responder). If off duty and responding voluntarily, the rescuer would generally be covered under the Good Samaritan Law.

Maintain your Skills: Review and practice your skills regularly; recertify every 2 years.

GOOD SAMARITAN LAW

Every state and nearly every country has a version of a Good Samaritan Law. Most states put this law in place in an effort to reduce the fear of being sued when providing care to an ill or injured patient. Research the law in your state.

The requirements for protection under the Good Samaritan Law usually include the following:

- Responding to a call for help or emergency situation on a voluntary basis.
- Not expecting compensation for rendering care.
- Providing care with common sense, reasonable skill and within the limits of your training.
- Not abandoning the patient after beginning care. Stay with the patient until help arrives.

GAINING CONSENT

The rescuer must obtain consent from the victim before beginning care. State your name and your level of training. Tell the victim what appears to be wrong and how you plan to help, then request permission to treat.

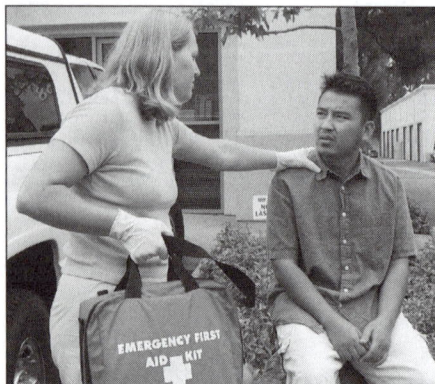

- **Expressed or Actual Consent –** The victim verbally expresses the desire for aid.

- **Implied Consent –** An unresponsive person cannot give consent; it is assumed.

- **Minor's Consent –** A parent or legal guardian must give consent before you begin care. If a parent or legal guardian is not present, and the condition is life threatening, treat the minor under implied consent.

Right to Privacy: Do not give the patient's information out to bystanders or coworkers. Keep private information private.

Refusal of Care: Every adult has the right to refuse treatment. An unresponsive patient may regain consciousness and refuse care. Call EMS (911) and have them evaluate the patient. When in doubt, it is best to begin care and activate EMS (call 911).

The Human Immunodeficiency Virus (HIV), Hepatitis B (HBV) and C (HCV), are viruses that are carried in the blood and body fluids of infected individuals. They are transmitted by the exchange of body fluids from person to person. Body fluids that are known to carry the infections are semen, vaginal secretions, saliva, cerebrospinal fluid, amniotic fluid, and any fluid visibly contaminated with blood.

At emergency scenes, treat all victims as potential carriers.

For a rescuer to be exposed, blood or body fluids from an infected individual must enter the rescuer's body.

Caution

Biohazard

- The easiest way for this to occur is through a **direct splash** on the rescuer's mucous membranes. Areas of concern are the eyes, mouth and nose.
- Another way for the rescuer to be exposed is by the virus entering through an **opening in the rescuer's skin.** The virus may enter through an open scab, a fresh cut, or a skin breakdown such as a rash.

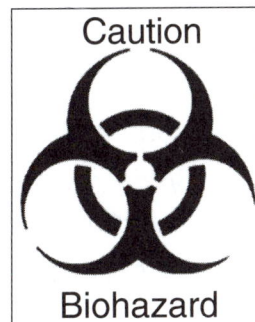

UNIVERSAL PRECAUTIONS

First responders must eliminate or minimize exposures by following **Universal Precautions** with all patients on every emergency scene. For additional protection, assume that all moist body substances are potentially infectious. Universal Precautions are as follows:

- Wash hands thoroughly before and after every patient contact.
- Use **Personal Protective Equipment** (moisture-proof disposable gloves, mask, gown, and eye protection). Put them on before starting treatment. Use non-latex gloves if possible.
- Use CPR barrier devices when providing rescue breathing.

Designated emergency responders should ask their employers about the availability of HBV vaccinations.

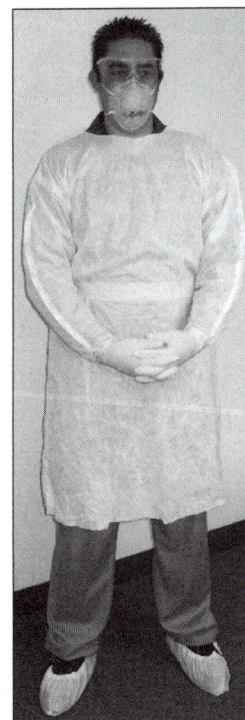

To remove soiled gloves:

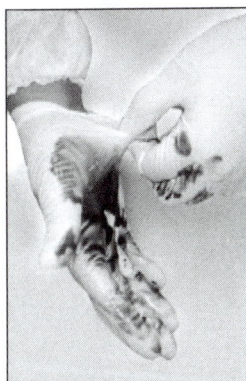

Pinch base of glove and peel off slowly.

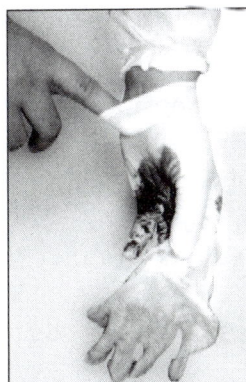

Place soiled glove in opposite hand; slip finger under glove and peel off.

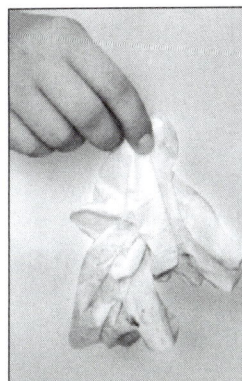

Finish so that gloves are inside out. Dispose of gloves properly.

An emergency is an unexpected occurrence that demands serious attention. Emergencies can happen anywhere and usually when you least expect them. Be prepared before one happens.

Pay attention to sights, sounds and situations that are unusual:

- Screams or panicked facial expressions
- A person who appears seriously ill or injured (e.g. clutching the chest, severe bleeding, facial or verbal expressions of pain)
- A collision or vehicle stopped in an unusual location
- A suspicious environment (e.g. overturned furniture or plants, opened chemical or medication containers, broken glass, blood)
- Environmental hazards (e.g. fire, explosion, damaged electrical wires, flooding)

The most important actions are to remain calm, stay aware of your own safety, and call 911.

DON'T DELAY CALLING 911

Statistics show that a person has a better chance of surviving an emergency when 911 is called early. Do not think someone else will call. Do not transport someone in your own car to the hospital.

When you call 911 or your local emergency response number:

- You are connected to a law enforcement or fire department/EMS dispatcher.
- While the dispatcher is talking with you, he or she is simultaneously sending help your way.
- Provide your name, location, and a description of the event.
- Always hang up last.

If your workplace has an internal medical response system, activate that system instead of calling 911 directly.

B.R.E.A.T.H.

Be safe when responding to an emergency.

Use the acronym **B.R.E.A.T.H.** to remind you of scene safety.

Be Prepared: First aid kit, CPR barrier device, training and retraining; carry a cell phone.

Relax: Take a moment to gather your thoughts and establish priorities.

Environment: Consider the hazards of the environment. Size up the scene before you act.

ABCD'S: Airway, Breathing, Compression, Defibrillation, Severe bleeding and Shock.

Treatment or Triage: Estimate the number of victims; focus on those who can be saved.

Help: Ensure help is on the way, and that someone knows what you are doing.

The cardiovascular system consists of the heart, blood vessels and blood. It is responsible for the delivery of oxygen and nutrients to the cells, and the removal of waste products such as carbon dioxide. The cardiovascular and respiratory systems work together in the lungs to exchange carbon dioxide for oxygen.

CARDIOVASCULAR SYSTEM

The heart is a hollow, muscular organ that is responsible for pumping blood throughout the body. It is about the size of your fist and is located in the center of your chest. Arteries are vessels that transport blood away from the heart to the tissues, while veins carry blood back to the heart. The coronary arteries provide a fresh supply of oxygenated blood to the heart muscle to keep it alive.

The heart is divided into four chambers. The chambers on top are the right and left atria; the chambers on the bottom are the right and left ventricles. When electrically stimulated, the atria contract and pump blood from the top of the heart to the ventricles below. The ventricles contract next and pump blood to the lungs and the body tissues. First the atria contract, then the ventricles.

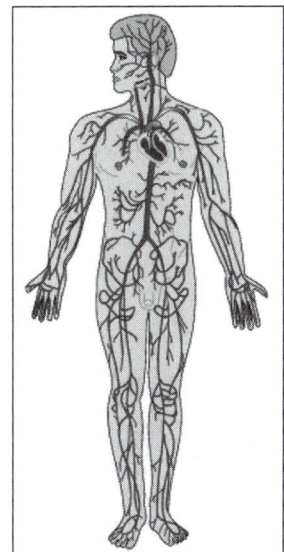

PHYSIOLOGY OF THE HEART

The pumping action of the heart is controlled by the heart's electrical conduction system. Unlike other muscles, its movement is stimulated by electrical impulses that originate from within. The electrical impulses are generated by a group of specialized cells called pacemakers. The chief **pacemaker** of the heart is the Sinoatrial (S-A) node, and is located in the right atrium.

During a heart attack, the heart muscle is deprived of oxygen. Cardiac cells in the affected area become irritated from the decreased supply of oxygen, and premature contractions begin to occur. As the heart works harder to obtain more oxygen, it demands more oxygen to compensate for the increased workload. A higher oxygen demand means more electrical impulses. As the heart is overloaded with electrical impulses, it may go into a rhythm known as **ventricular fibrillation** (V-Fib) in which the heart stops beating and there is no circulation. V-Fib is the most common initial rhythm associated with witnessed SCA.

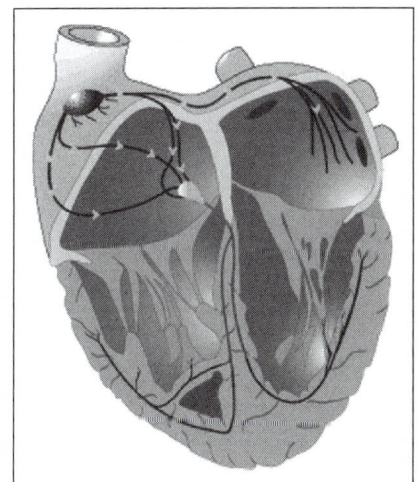

Pacemaker cells generate a heartbeat.

Fat and cholesterol are contained in many of the foods we eat. Cholesterol is carried by the blood and may attach to the walls of the coronary arteries. Over time, plaque and cholesterol buildup causes narrowing of the coronary arteries **(atherosclerosis)**, and may result in a complete blockage.

A **heart attack** occurs when a fat or blood clot blocks a narrowed coronary artery, depriving the heart muscle of oxygen. The heart attack victim feels discomfort because the heart muscle is dying. Heart attack is the leading cause of sudden cardiac arrest.

CARDIAC RISK FACTORS

Controllable Risk Factors	Methods of Prevention*	Non-Controllable Risk Factors
Decreased physical activity	Exercise: Cardiovascular, at least 3 times/week	
High blood pressure	Exercise, medication, diet	Age
High blood cholesterol	Exercise, medication, diet	Family History
Diabetes	Careful regulation of blood sugar levels, medication	Male
Obesity/Diet	Healthy, varied, low-fat diet	Post-menopausal Female
Stress	Exercise, relaxation techniques, rest, reduce life stressors	
Smoking	Quit	

*Do not begin an exercise program or changes in lifestyle without first consulting a physician.

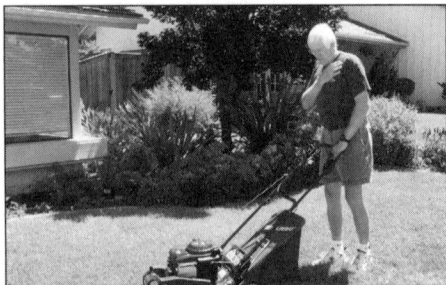

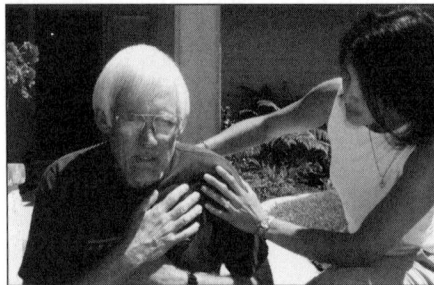

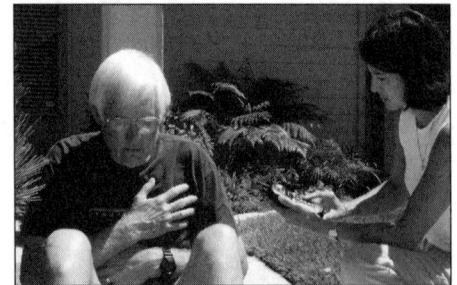

SIGNS AND SYMPTOMS:

The warning signs of a heart attack may come in any combination. If any of the following signs or symptoms are present for five minutes, call 911.

* Chest discomfort: pain, pressure, tightness, squeezing, fullness. May radiate to arms, neck, back or jaw, or may go away and return. May be mistaken for heartburn or indigestion.

* Pale, cool, moist (sweaty) skin

* Shortness of breath

* Dizziness or fainting

* Nausea or vomiting

* Denial: Ignoring or attributing symptoms of heart attack to another cause.

TREATMENT:

1. Recognize the signs and symptoms of possible heart attack.
2. Place in a position of comfort; rest and reassure. Do not lay the patient down unless unresponsive, dizzy or faint.
3. Help patient locate and self-administer prescribed medication, usually nitro-glycerin.
4. If discomfort persists for five minutes, activate EMS. Do not delay.
5. If the patient becomes unresponsive:
   a. Send a bystander to call 911 (or go call if alone) and get the AED.
   b. ABCD'S

Note: Women, diabetics, and the elderly may not have the typical symptom of chest discomfort. Be alert to other symptoms, such as extreme fatigue, nausea, vomiting, or shortness of breath. Women are as likely to have a heart attack as men, but are less often diagnosed correctly.

The brain is the nerve center for the body. Its signals are sent through electrical currents that travel down the body's nervous system. These impulses from the brain control nearly every aspect of the body. The brain relies on oxygen and sugar. Like the heart, it is fed nutrients through a system of blood vessels. When one of those vessels becomes obstructed (blockage) or ruptures (bleed), the flow of blood is disrupted and brain cells begin to die.

A **cerebrovascular accident (CVA)**, or **stroke**, occurs when oxygen-rich blood is unable to reach a portion of the brain. This may be due to a ruptured blood vessel or a traveling clot.

A **transient ischemic attack (TIA)** is a temporary lack of oxygen with total recovery of function. It may last a few seconds or several hours. A TIA may be a warning sign of a future stroke. Contact a doctor for evaluation.

TYPES OF STROKE

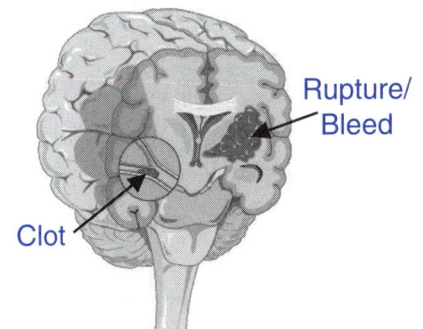

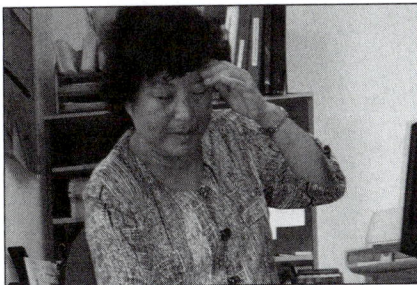

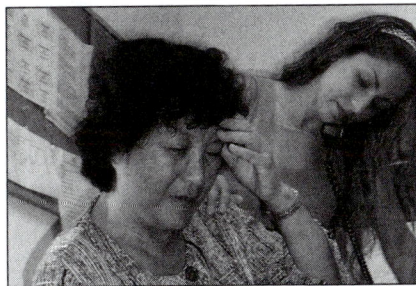

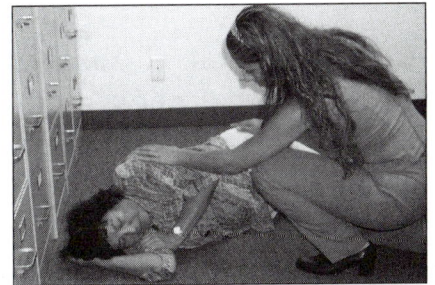

Rupture/Bleed

Clot

SIGNS & SYMPTOMS (SUDDEN ONSET):
- Decreased mental status
- Facial droop and drooling
- Weakness in arms and legs (usually on one side of the body)
- Slurred speech or inability to speak
- Loss of balance or coordination
- Difficulty swallowing
- Changes in sensation
- Headache, blurred vision

TREATMENT:
1. ABCD'S
2. Protect airway.
3. Reassure patient.
4. Activate EMS system.
5. Perform patient assessment.
6. If unresponsive, place in the recovery position on the affected side to allow fluids to drain.

A stroke is a serious medical emergency. The time it takes for a patient to reach the hospital is a major factor in determining recovery. Clot busting medications are only effective in the early hours of a stroke and may be withheld if the patient does not reach the emergency department soon enough.

Tip: Use **STR** to quickly look for common signs of a stroke:

Smile: Ask patient to smile. Both sides of the face should move equally.

Talk: Ask patient to repeat a common phrase. Listen for slurred or incorrect words.

Reach: Ask patient to close eyes and raise arms. Look for arm drift or weakness on one side.

The goal of **CPR (cardiopulmonary resuscitation)** is to provide oxygenated blood flow to the brain to keep it alive, and to the heart to increase the chance for successful defibrillation.

When a person suffers from respiratory arrest (no breathing) and cardiac arrest (no heartbeat), the brain is not receiving oxygen. Without oxygen, brain cells begin to die, causing irreversible brain damage within 4 to 6 minutes. After 10 minutes, all brain cells are dead. CPR combines external chest compressions with rescue breathing to provide oxygen to the brain.

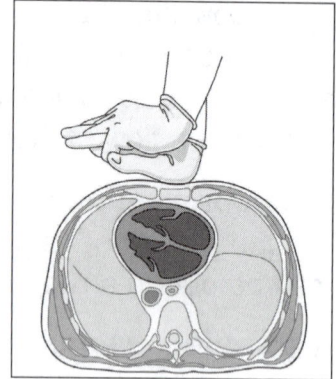

HOW DOES CPR WORK?

Artificial respiration **(rescue breathing)** provides oxygen to the patient's lungs. External **chest compressions** squeeze the heart between the sternum (breastbone) and the spine. As the chest is compressed, blood is forced from the heart to the lungs, where it picks up oxygen. When pressure is released, the heart refills with blood. The oxygenated blood is delivered to the body tissues through continuous chest compressions. CPR is about 30% as effective as a heart beating on its own.

Chest compressions must be performed correctly, with minimal interruptions, and on a firm surface to be effective.

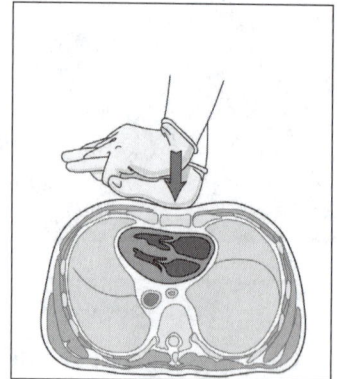

WHAT ELSE CAN I DO?

In sudden cardiac arrest, CPR is used to provide oxygen, but will not restore the victim's circulation. The heart of an adult cardiac arrest victim usually requires an electrical shock to beat normally again. A shockable state only exists for a few minutes after SCA.

The **automated external defibrillator (AED)** enables first responders to provide defibrillation prior to the arrival of EMS personnel. When early defibrillation is combined with effective CPR, a victim's chance of survival is dramatically increased.

AEDs are commonly seen at airports, stadiums, sporting events, shopping malls, golf courses, schools, and many public venues.

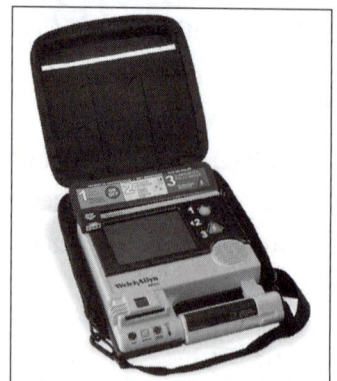

The AED is a computerized device that can evaluate a person's heart rhythm. If it recognizes a rhythm that requires a shock, it can deliver the shock. It is very simple and safe to use, and will not incorrectly discharge an electrical shock.

The AED provides the user with simple directions through voice prompts and visual indicators. Without immediate AED use, the CPR survival rate is approximately 5%. When an AED is used together with CPR immediately after collapse, the survival rate can be as high as 74%!

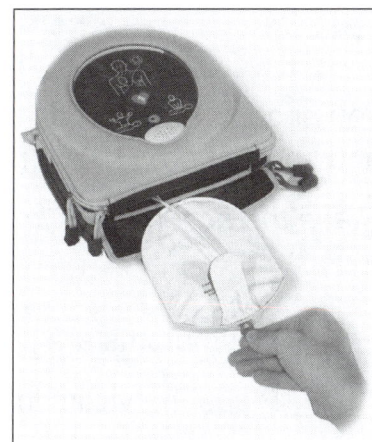

AED

STOPPING VENTRICULAR FIBRILLATION

In sudden cardiac arrest, the heart stops beating and is overwhelmed with chaotic electrical activity known as **ventricular fibrillation**. There is no circulation. Although CPR can supply fresh oxygen to the brain and vital organs to keep them alive, it cannot restore a heartbeat in the adult patient. CPR buys time until a defibrillator arrives.

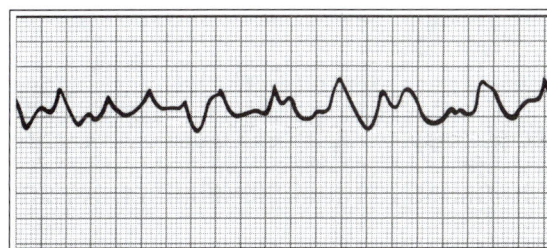

V-Fib

Defibrillation is the only way to stop the chaotic electrical impulses and correct ventricular fibrillation. The sooner a shock from a defibrillator is given, the better the chance of restoring the heart to a normal rhythm.

DEFIBRILLATION

A defibrillator runs a rapid, powerful electrical current through the heart, resulting in a brief pause of the heart's electrical activity. This allows the heart to resume its normal electrical rhythm, hopefully creating a muscular contraction (heartbeat).

An AED can be used by lay providers and professional rescuers for both adults and children before the arrival of the paramedics. It's important to be familiar with the location and operation of the AED at your workplace. An AED should be used within 3 - 5 minutes of cardiac arrest for the best outcome.

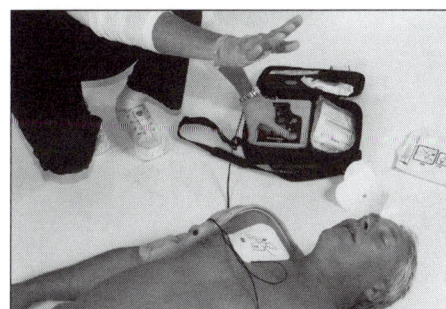

You encounter a woman in the store who is clutching her chest and shoulder, and appears sweaty and short of breath. You recognize these signs and symptoms of possible heart attack.

Place the action steps in correct sequence.

_____ If symptoms are present for 5 minutes, ask a bystander to activate the EMS system.

_____ Place the victim in a position of comfort, usually sitting up. Reassure the victim.

_____ Help the patient self-administer nitroglycerin.

_____ Introduce yourself, state that you are trained in first aid, and ask for permission to help her.

An employee provides first aid to a bleeding co-worker. After he finishes cleaning the blood spill, he notices that his glove is ripped, and that his co-worker's blood has entered a cut.

Place the action steps in correct sequence.

_____ Report the exposure to the supervisor.

_____ Remove soiled PPE and dispose of in proper container.

_____ Wash hands thoroughly with soap and warm water, and bandage the cut.

The **ABCD'S** are a series of actions a rescuer takes to determine if an unresponsive patient's **A**irway is open, if he or she is **B**reathing, if **C**ompressions and **D**efibrillation are needed, and if the patient is bleeding **S**everely or in **S**hock. Before performing the ABCD'S, attempt to establish a response from the patient.

Establish Responsiveness: Put on gloves, tap the shoulders and shout at the patient.

If the patient does not respond:

- Shout for help and send a bystander to activate EMS and get the AED.

If alone:

- For an unresponsive **adult**, activate EMS and get the AED *before* performing the ABCD'S.
- For an unresponsive **child or infant**, activate EMS and get the AED (child) *after* performing the ABCD'S and 2 minutes of CPR.

Log roll a victim who is face down onto his or her back.

A – OPEN THE AIRWAY

The airway extends from the lips to the lungs. When a patient becomes unresponsive, the tongue relaxes, falling back in the throat and covering the trachea (windpipe). **The tongue is the most common cause of airway obstruction in the unresponsive patient.** A patient may begin to breathe again when a rescuer opens the airway, lifting the tongue off the back of the throat.

Open the airway with the **head tilt/chin lift maneuver.**

1. Place one hand on the forehead. Place 2 or 3 fingers on the bony part of the jaw.

2. Lift the chin up while tilting the head back.

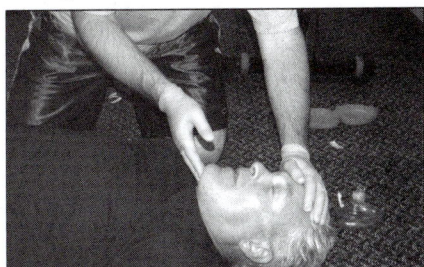

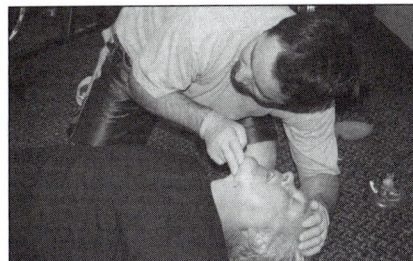

B – CHECK FOR BREATHING

While maintaining an open airway, place your head near the patient's face with your ear near his or her mouth. Look, listen and feel for breathing for 5 - 10 seconds.

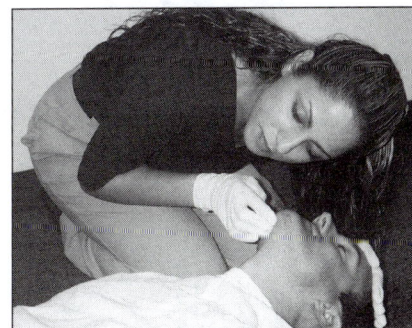

Look for chest movement.

Listen for sounds of breathing.

Feel with your cheek and ear for air flow or warmth.

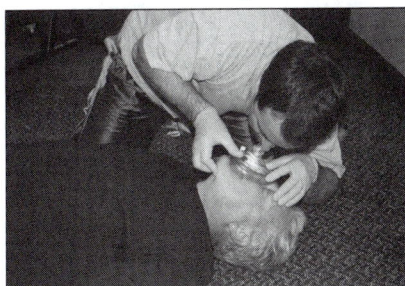

If the patient is not breathing normally (adult), give 2 rescue breaths.

- For 1 second each.
- Just enough for chest rise.

Adult: Gasping or irregular breathing is not normal breathing.

Child or Infant: Check for the presence of any breathing.

C – Chest Compressions

If an unresponsive patient is not breathing, give 2 rescue breaths, then quickly remove clothing from the front of the chest that may interfere with compressions. Immediately begin **compressions**.

- **Rate** – 100 compressions per minute
- **Depth** –
  - **Adult**: 1½ - 2 inches
  - **Child and Infant**: $1/3$ to $1/2$ the depth of the chest
- **Location** –
  - **Adult and Child**: Center of the chest between the nipples
  - **Infant**: Just below the nipple line
- **Ratio** – 30 compressions to 2 ventilations (30:2)
- Perform 5 cycles of 30:2 in 2 minutes.
- Allow full chest recoil.
- Decrease interruptions to compressions.

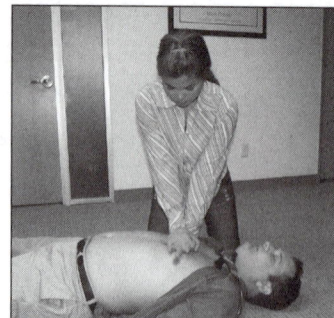

PRESS FIRM AND FAST

D – Defibrillation

An AED should be ready to deliver a shock within 90 seconds of its arrival. If a second trained rescuer is present, continue CPR while the AED is prepared for use.

1. Turn on the AED.
2. Apply pads to chest; attach connector cables if needed.
3. Stop CPR to allow the AED to analyze the heart rhythm.
4. Press shock button if prompted.
5. Immediately resume CPR, beginning with chest compressions.
6. Follow additional AED prompts.
7. If no shock is advised, continue CPR as needed.

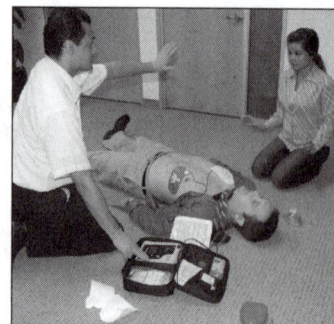

Coordinate CPR with AED use to minimize interruptions to compressions. The shorter the time between chest compressions, shock delivery, and resumption of compressions, the more likely the shock will succeed.

S – Severe Bleeding/Shock

If breathing normally:

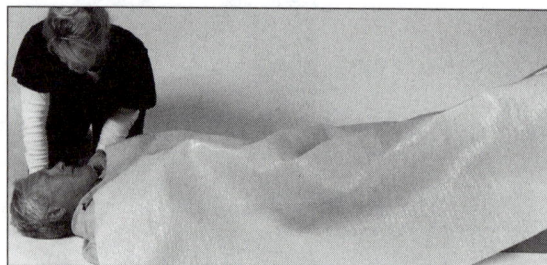

Treat the patient for **Shock** by raising the legs and keeping the patient warm.

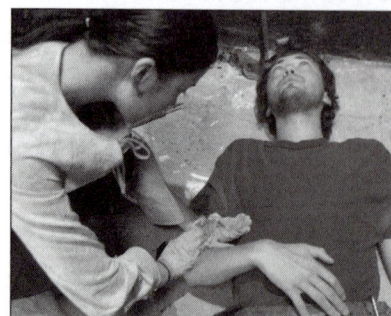

Control **Severe bleeding** with the use of direct pressure.

During most emergency situations, a victim should be left as found until professional rescuers arrive. **Only move a patient if he or she is in immediate danger, has a compromised airway, or requires a firm, flat surface for CPR.**

The recovery position helps a rescuer manage an unresponsive patient by maintaining an open airway and allowing fluids to drain. Use the recovery position:

- When an unresponsive victim is breathing normally.
- When an unresponsive victim begins moving after CPR, AED, or choking episode.
- When a rescuer needs to leave an unresponsive person to summon help.

The recovery position is not recommended for infants or small children, because it may obstruct the airway if the head is not supported.

Log Roll

Use the **log roll** technique to place a victim in the recovery position.

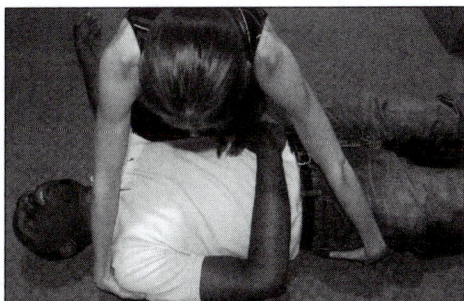

1.
Grasp the hip and shoulder furthest from you and roll the victim towards you, keeping the head, neck and back in line.

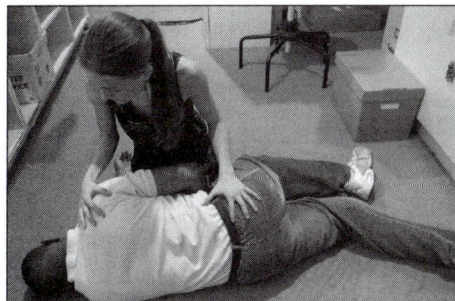

2.
Place the victim on his or her side, with the lower arm in front. Bend one or both knees and make other small adjustments to make sure the victim can remain in the recovery position unassisted.

If a **neck or back injury** is suspected:

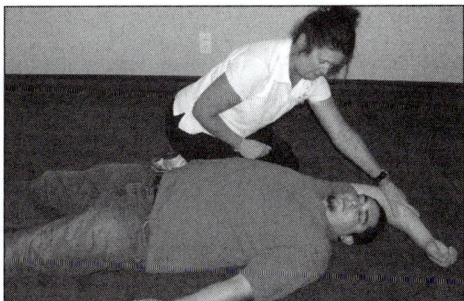

1.
Grasp the arm closest to you and gently lift it over the top of the head. Roll the victim towards you, keeping the head, neck and back in line.

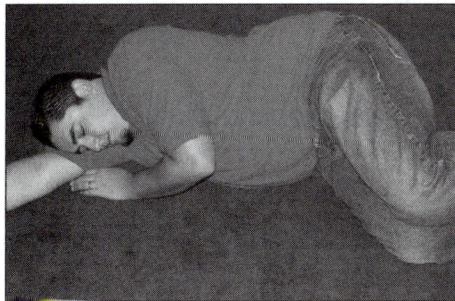

2.
When the victim is on his or her side, the head will be supported by the raised arm. Bend both knees to stabilize the victim.

Continue to monitor breathing. Be ready to start CPR.

A victim who is **obviously pregnant** should be placed on her left side to avoid complications caused by the weight of the baby pressing down on vital blood vessels.

ESTABLISH RESPONSIVENESS

Assessment: Is the patient responsive or unresponsive?

- Tap and shout at the patient.

Action: Activate EMS.

- If unresponsive, shout for help and send a bystander to call 911 and get the AED.
- If alone, go call 911, get the AED and return to the patient as quickly as possible.
- Ensure the victim is on a firm, flat surface.

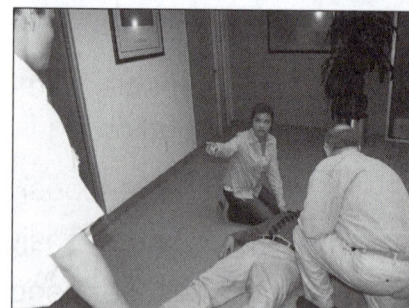

Establish response, send bystander to call 911.

A: AIRWAY

Assessment: Is the airway open?

Action: Open the airway with the head tilt/chin lift.

> The tongue is the most common cause of airway obstruction in the unresponsive person. Proper positioning of the head prevents the tongue from blocking the airway.

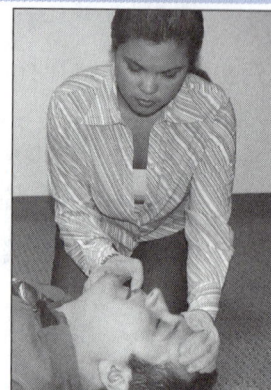

Head tilt/chin lift

B: BREATHING

Assessment: Is the victim breathing normally?

- Maintain an open airway with the head tilt/chin lift.
- Look, listen and feel for normal breathing for 5 - 10 seconds.
  - ◆ Occasional gasping or irregular breathing is not normal breathing.

Action: Give 2 rescue breaths.

- Pinch nose and seal victim's mouth with yours.
- 1 second each breath.
- Ensure chest rises with each breath.
- Do not over-ventilate.
- If no chest rise, reposition the head and give a second breath.
- Immediately begin chest compressions.

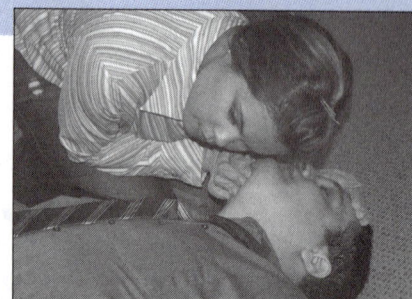

Look, listen and feel for breathing for 5-10 seconds.

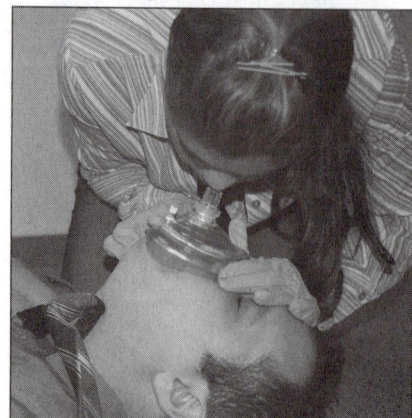

Give 2 breaths.

C: Compression

Assessment: None

Action: Begin chest compressions.

- Quickly remove clothing from the front of the chest that may interfere with compressions.
- Place the heel of one hand on the lower half of the sternum between the nipples.
- Place the other hand on top of the first, keeping the fingers lifted off the chest wall (rib area).
- Using the heel of your hand, compress the chest 30 times.
  - Depth: 1$\frac{1}{2}$ - 2 inches
  - Rate: 100/minute
  - Allow full chest recoil.

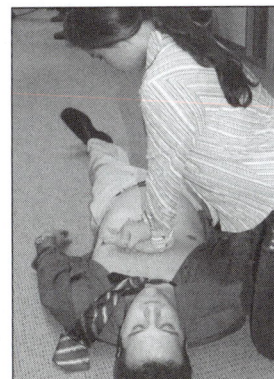

PRESS FIRM and FAST

Continue CPR without stopping.

- Cycles of 30 chest compressions followed by 2 breaths (30:2).
- Decrease interruptions to compressions.
- If the victim vomits, log roll him/her, clear the airway, return to back, and continue CPR.
- If a trained bystander is present, rotate rescuers every 2 minutes.

D: Defibrillation

Assessment: Is the AED ready and the scene safe?
- Patient is not in a puddle of water.
- No free-flowing oxygen present.

| See pages 22 - 28 for detailed AED information. |

Action: Use the AED.

- Turn on the AED and follow the prompts.
- Expose the chest and wipe dry.
- Apply pads; connect to AED.
- Follow AED prompts.
  - Stop CPR, clear the patient, and allow the AED to analyze the rhythm.
  - If prompted to shock:
    - Ensure no one is touching the patient: "I'm clear, you're clear, we're all clear"
    - Press shock button.
- Resume CPR, starting with compressions.
- Follow additional AED prompts. If no shock advised, continue CPR as needed.

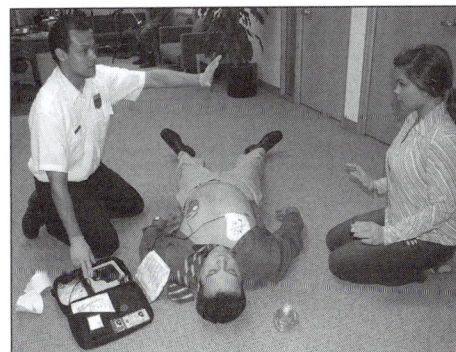

If the victim begins to move, leave the AED pads in place. Maintain an open airway or place victim in the recovery position; monitor breathing. Be ready to start CPR if needed.

Cardiac arrest in children usually occurs as a result of **respiratory arrest**.

Respiratory arrest in children is often caused by:

- Traumatic injury
- Poisoning
- Drowning
- Choking
- Respiratory illness
  (e.g. asthma, pneumonia)

When a child is unable to breathe, the heart rate will begin to slow and eventually stop. By providing CPR to a child, the rescuer may be able to restore normal circulation without the use of an AED. However, the rescuer should still bring an AED to the scene of a child in cardiac arrest. The lone rescuer should provide CPR for 2 minutes before leaving to call 911.

ESTABLISH RESPONSIVENESS

Assessment: Is the patient responsive or unresponsive?
- Tap and shout at the patient.

Action: Activate EMS.
- If unresponsive, shout for help and send a bystander to call 911 and get the AED.
- If alone, begin CPR if indicated.
- Ensure the child is on a firm, flat surface.

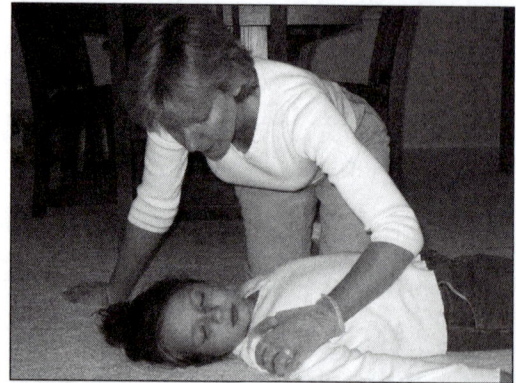

A: AIRWAY

Assessment: Is the airway open?

Action: Open the airway with the head tilt/chin lift.

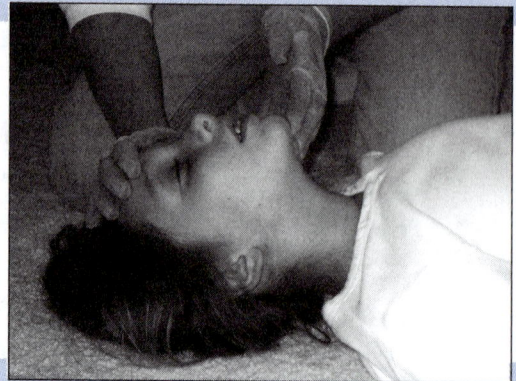

B: BREATHING

Assessment: Is the victim breathing?
- Maintain an open airway with the head tilt/chin lift.
- Look, listen and feel for breathing for 5 - 10 seconds.

Action: Give 2 rescue breaths.
- Pinch nose and seal victim's mouth with yours.
- 1 second each breath.
- Ensure chest rises with each breath.
- Do not over-ventilate.
- If no chest rise, reposition the head and give a second breath.
- Immediately begin chest compressions.

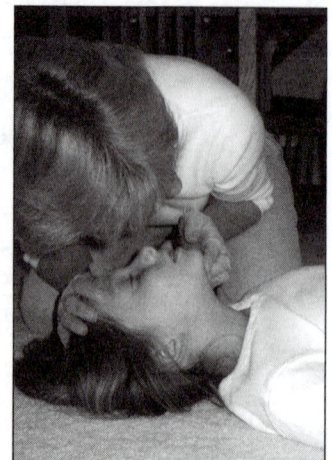

C: COMPRESSION

Assessment: None

Action: Begin chest compressions.

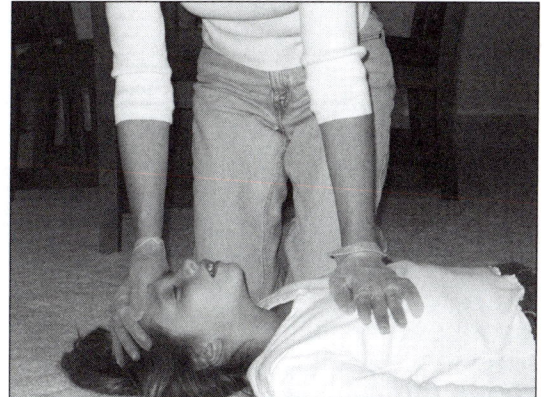

- Quickly remove clothing from the front of the chest that may interfere with compressions.
- Place the heel of one hand on the lower half of the sternum between the nipples, keeping the fingers lifted off the chest wall.
- Keep the airway open with your other hand on the forehead.
- Using the heel of your hand, compress the chest 30 times.
    - Depth: $1/3$ to $1/2$ the depth of the chest.
    - Rate: 100/minute
    - Allow full chest recoil.
- Use 2 hands for compression if needed to reach adequate depth.

Continue CPR for 2 minutes.

- 5 cycles of 30:2
- Call 911 if not previously contacted, and quickly return to continue CPR.
- Decrease interruptions to compressions.
- If the child vomits, log roll him or her, clear the airway, return to back, and continue CPR.
- If a trained bystander is present, rotate rescuers every 2 minutes.

D: DEFIBRILLATION

Assessment: Is the AED ready and the scene safe?
- Patient is not in a puddle of water.
- No free-flowing oxygen present.

Action: Use the AED after about 2 minutes of CPR.
- Turn on the AED and follow the prompts.
- Expose the chest and wipe dry.
- Apply pads; connect to AED.
    - Use pediatric pads or equipment, if available.
- Follow AED prompts.
    - Stop CPR, clear the patient, and allow the AED to analyze the rhythm.
    - If prompted to shock:
        - Ensure no one is touching the patient: "I'm clear, you're clear, we're all clear."
        - Press shock button.
- Resume CPR, starting with compressions.
- Follow additional AED prompts. If no shock advised, continue CPR as needed.

See pages 22 - 28 for detailed AED information.

For the purpose of defibrillation, a child is considered to be age 1 - 8, or weigh < 55 lbs.

Cardiac arrest in infants, as in children, usually occurs after breathing has stopped.

Respiratory arrest in infants is often caused by:

- Traumatic injury
- SIDS
- Drowning
- Choking
- Respiratory illness (e.g. asthma, pneumonia)

Lack of oxygen causes the infant's heart to slow and eventually stop. By providing CPR to an infant, the rescuer may be able to restore normal circulation without the use of advanced techniques. The lone rescuer should provide CPR for 2 minutes before leaving to call 911.

ESTABLISH RESPONSIVENESS

Assessment: Is the patient responsive or unresponsive?
- Tap and shout, flick the soles of the feet.

Action: Activate EMS.
- If unresponsive, shout for help and send a bystander to call 911.
- If alone, begin CPR if indicated.
- Ensure the infant is on a firm, flat surface. Use a table if available.

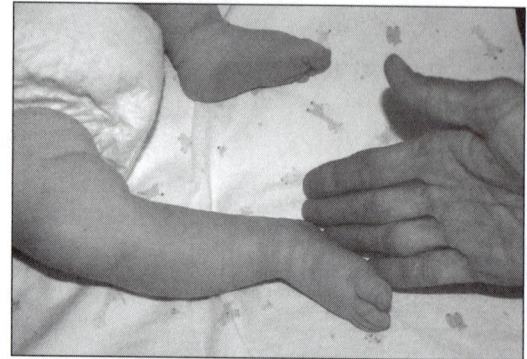

A: AIRWAY

Assessment: Is the airway open?

Action: Open the airway with the head tilt/chin lift.
- **Keep the infant's head in a neutral position.**
- Hyperextension of the neck can obstruct the airway of an infant.

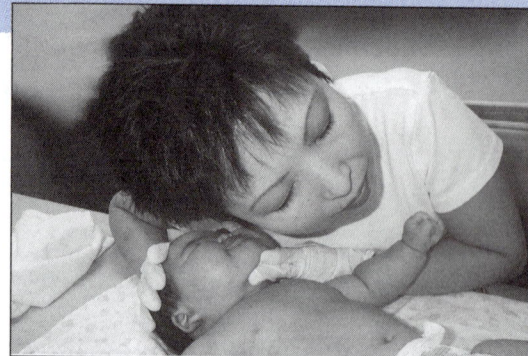

B: BREATHING

Assessment: Is the victim breathing?
- Maintain an open airway with the head tilt/chin lift.
- Look, listen and feel for breathing for 5 - 10 seconds.

Action: Give 2 rescue breaths.
- Seal victim's **mouth and nose** with your mouth.
- 1 second each breath.
- Ensure chest rises with each breath.
- Do not over-ventilate.
- If rescuer cannot cover victim's mouth and nose, attempt mouth-to-mouth or mouth-to-nose rescue breathing.
- If no chest rise, reposition the head and give a second breath.
- Immediately begin chest compressions.

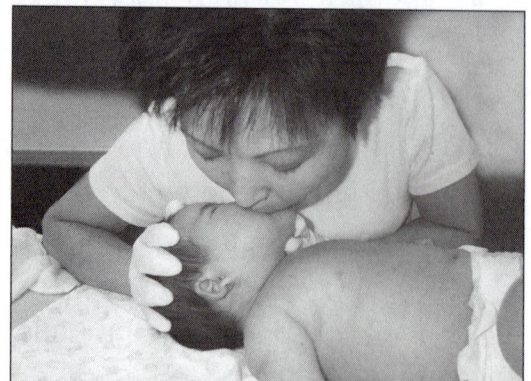

Assessment: None

Action: Begin chest compressions.

- Quickly remove clothing from the front of the chest that may interfere with compressions.
- Place 2 fingers in the center of the chest just below the nipple line.
- Keep the airway open with your other hand on the forehead.
- Using 2 fingers, compress the chest 30 times.
  - Depth: $1/3$ to $1/2$ the depth of the chest.
  - Rate: 100/minute
  - Allow full chest recoil.

Continue CPR for 2 minutes.

- 5 cycles of 30:2
- Call 911 if not previously contacted, and return to the patient as quickly as possible.
- Continue CPR as needed.
- Decrease interruptions to compressions.
- If the infant vomits, log roll him/her, clear the airway, return to back, and continue CPR.

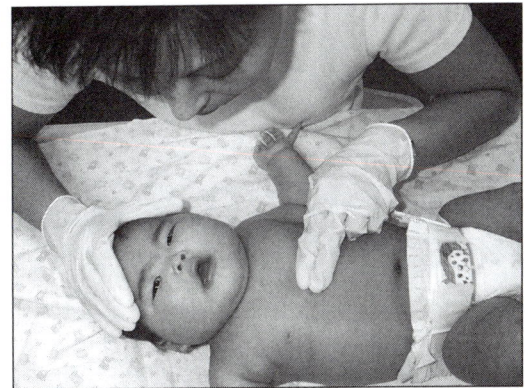

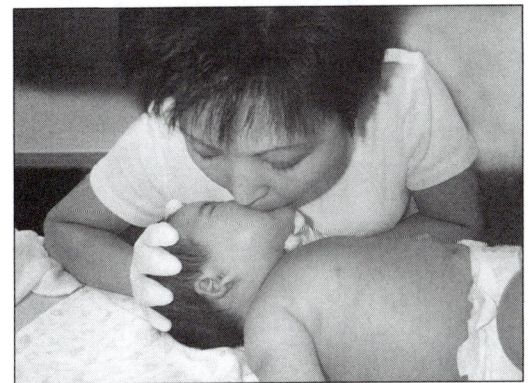

If the infant begins to move, maintain an open airway; monitor breathing. Be ready to start CPR if needed. The recovery position is not recommended for infants or small children, because it may obstruct the airway if the head is not supported.

Should I carry the baby to the phone?

If a lone rescuer has performed CPR for 2 minutes on a small child or infant and trauma has NOT occurred, consider carrying the victim with you to a phone to contact EMS more quickly. If a second rescuer is present, send him or her to call EMS.

No recommendation at this time.

An AED should be kept in an accessible area, close to a phone. **If you are locking up the AED, be sure that every trained rescuer has a key**. Store an AED at room temperature, protected from the elements. Follow manufacturer's guidelines for storage.

The AED should be charged and ready for use. Accessories such as extra pads, pediatric pads or adaptor, an extra battery, CPR barrier masks, a towel, gloves and razor should be stored with the AED. Perform inspection and testing according to manufacturer's guidelines. Ensure that expiration dates are current, and there is no visible damage.

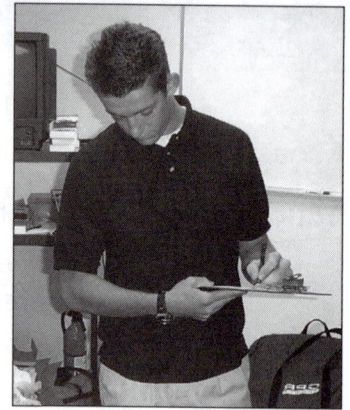

Troubleshooting: If the unit identifies a problem during AED use, it will prompt you to troubleshoot the problem. AED troubleshooting prompts can include:

- **Check the pads:** Press down firmly or replace with new pads; check cable connection.
- **Low battery:** Replace the battery.
- **Patient movement:** When the AED is analyzing the heart rhythm, do not touch or move the patient (i.e. stop the gurney or vehicle; "clear" the patient).

AED PADS

Pad Placement: Expose the chest of the victim and wipe dry of any moisture. Peel off the backing and apply the sticky side of the pad according to the picture on the pad. Apply one pad to the right upper chest, and the other pad to the lower left side of the chest. Pad placement may be varied to accommodate implanted devices or other needs.

Children: Children age 1 - 8 or weighing less than 55 lbs. require a smaller electrical shock to defibrillate the heart. This can be accomplished through the use of special child pads, or an energy reducer or switch for the AED. If pediatric-specific electrode pads or equipment is unavailable, adult pads can be used.

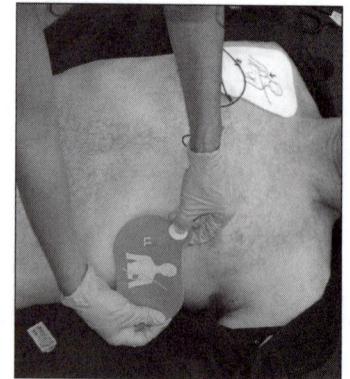

CLEARING THE PATIENT

It is critical that no one is touching the patient when the AED analyzes or delivers a shock. When prompted by the AED to shock the patient:

- The rescuer using the AED will hold his or her arm out over the patient, look down at his/her own body and loudly state, "I'm clear."
- He or she will look up and down the entire patient, ensure that no one else is touching the patient, and loudly state, "You're clear. We're all clear."
- The rescuer can now press the shock button.

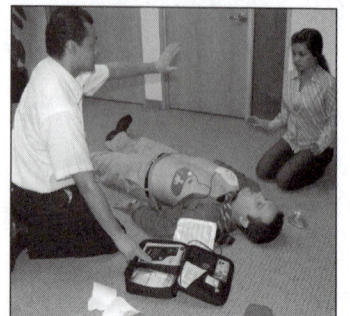

A **CPR barrier device** protects the rescuer from exposure to the blood or body fluids of the patient while giving rescue breaths. In some cases, barrier devices provide more effective ventilation than regular mouth-to-mouth breathing.

Face masks and face shields are transparent so that the rescuer can observe the mouth and nose during rescue breathing.

Face Mask

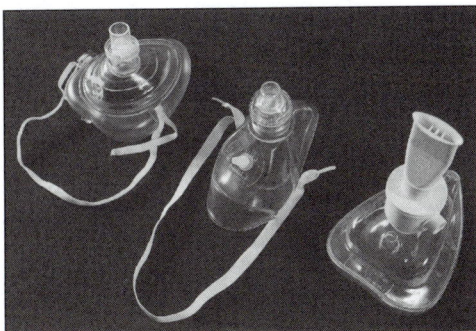

A **face mask** is a molded, mask-like plastic piece designed to fit over the mouth and nose of a patient. A one-way valve directs air into the patient, and directs exhaled air away from the rescuer. It will not allow blood or body fluids to escape into the mouth of the rescuer.

Some face masks come with an oxygen inlet to allow for supplemental oxygen administration. Select the correct size mask (adult, child or infant) to obtain an adequate seal.

1. Apply the mask so that the narrow portion is over the bridge of the nose, not covering the eyes. The bottom portion should not extend past the chin.
2. Create a seal by holding the top and bottom portions of the mask tightly to the face while lifting the chin into the open airway position.
3. Breathe into the mask as you would the patient's mouth; watch for chest rise.

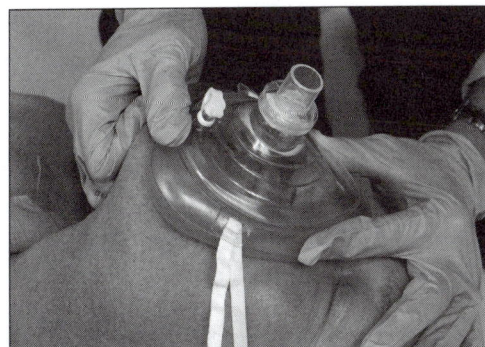

Note: If a pediatric mask is unavailable, rotate an adult mask so that the narrow end is over the mouth.

Face Shield

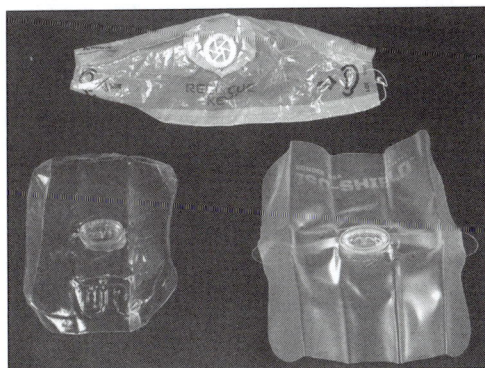

A **face shield** is a watertight plastic shield that contains a built-in one-way valve and/or filter.

1. Place the plastic shield over the victim's face with the valve over the mouth.
2. Pinch the victim's nose (over or under the face shield per manufacturer's guidelines).
3. Breathe into the one-way valve. Observe for chest rise and fall.

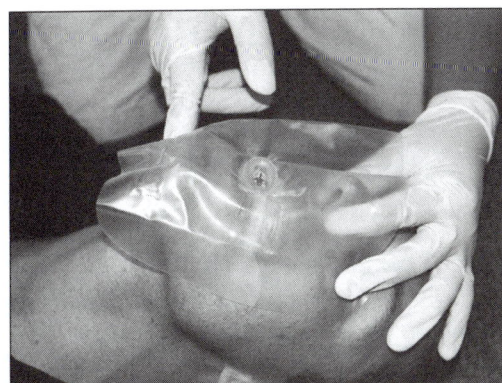

1. Ensure the environment is safe before beginning treatment.
2. Always use Universal Precautions:
   - Gloves, goggles, CPR barrier device, hand washing
3. Start CPR immediately after collapse.
   - Send a bystander to call 911 if available.
   - If alone with an **adult** victim, call 911 and get the AED *before* beginning CPR.
   - If alone with a **child** victim, call 911 and get the AED *after* 5 cycles of CPR.
4. Assess an **adult** victim for **normal breathing**.
   - Occasional gasping or irregular breathing is not normal breathing.

   Assess a **child or infant** victim for the presence of **any breathing**.
5. Chest compressions:
   - Perform CPR on a firm, flat surface.
   - Quickly remove clothing from the front of the chest that may interfere with compressions.
   - Press firm and fast. Compressions must be deep and fast enough to be effective.
   - Allow full chest recoil.
   - Decrease interruptions to compressions.
   - Perform compressions directly over the victim at a 90° angle, not from the side.
   - Chest compressions may fracture ribs. DO NOT stop CPR. Reassess hand position and continue.
6. If vomiting occurs, log roll the victim to the side, sweep out the mouth and continue CPR.

   To Avoid Vomiting:
   - Maintain an open airway when ventilating to avoid air entering the stomach.
   - Give each rescue breath for only 1 second.
   - Provide just enough air to obtain chest rise; do not over-inflate the lungs.
   - Allow the patient to exhale by removing your mouth from the patient's between breaths.
7. An AED will shock no more than once every 2 minutes. After delivering a shock, immediately resume CPR, beginning with compressions.
8. Do not remove AED pads from the patient.

DO NOT STOP CPR

Do not stop to reassess or move the patient.

Only stop CPR:
- When the patient begins to move.
- When professional rescuers take over.
- To use an AED.
- If you are physically exhausted and cannot continue.
- If the scene becomes unsafe.
- If the victim is pronounced dead by a qualified person.

Compression-Only CPR

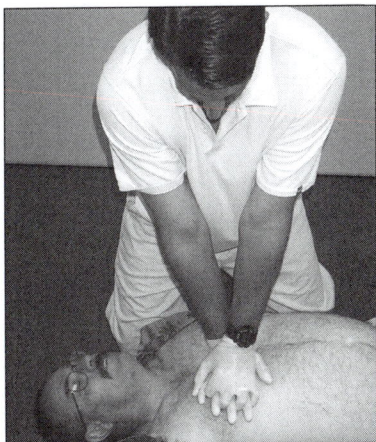

A victim will have the best chance of survival if both ventilations and compressions are provided. When a rescuer is unwilling or unable to provide ventilations, the patient can still benefit from compression-only CPR (without rescue breathing).

Mouth-to-Stoma Breathing

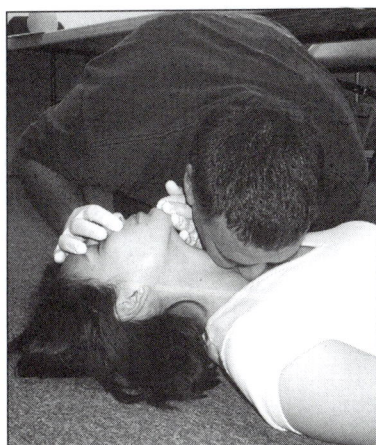

If the patient has a stoma (a surgically created opening at the base of the throat to allow for breathing), the rescuer will check for breathing with his or her ear above the stoma. If there is not adequate breathing, provide breaths through the stoma. Pinch the nose and close the patient's mouth to reduce air loss.

Mouth-to-Nose Breathing

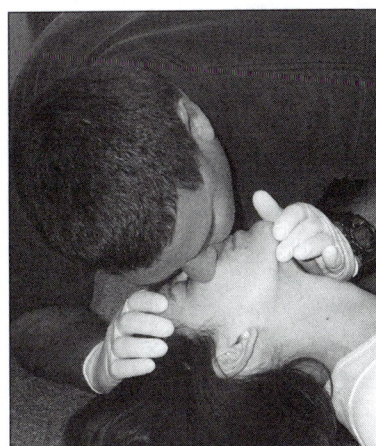

A rescuer may have to perform mouth-to-nose rescue breathing if a patient's mouth or jaw is severely damaged. Be sure to **hold the victim's mouth closed** so that air does not escape. During mouth-to-nose rescue breathing, lift your mouth from the victim's nose to allow passive exhalation.

When used properly, an AED presents no risk to the rescuers, bystanders and patients. Before using an AED, consider the environment and the surface on which the victim is lying. There are circumstances in which the user of the AED must take precautions.

Do Not Touch the Patient

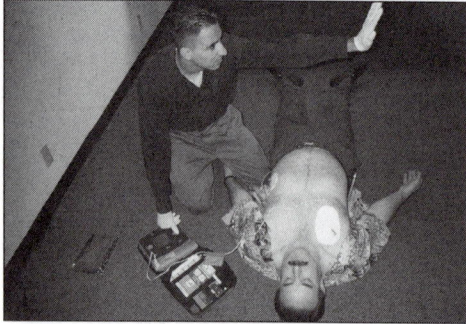

When an AED is analyzing or charged and ready to shock, make sure that no one is touching the patient or his or her clothes prior to delivering the shock. Look up and down the patient as you announce loudly, "I'm clear. You're clear. We're all clear."

What's wrong with this picture?

Water

Water is a great conductor of electricity. Move a patient who is lying in a puddle or pool of water to a drier area prior to AED use. Defibrillating a patient who is lying in water could cause burning or shocking to rescuers or bystanders. Ensure that the rescuer or bystanders are not standing in water during AED use. Rain, snow, or small amounts of water will not interfere with safe AED use.

Water or sweat on a victim's chest can interfere with defibrillation. Quickly dry the victim's chest before attaching the pads to ensure that the pads attach securely, and that the electrical shock travels through the heart and not over the wet surface of the skin.

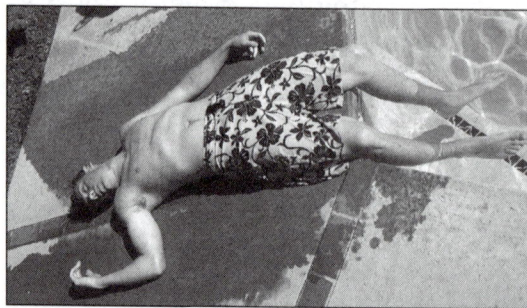

Remove a patient completely from the pool prior to using an AED.

Combustible Environment

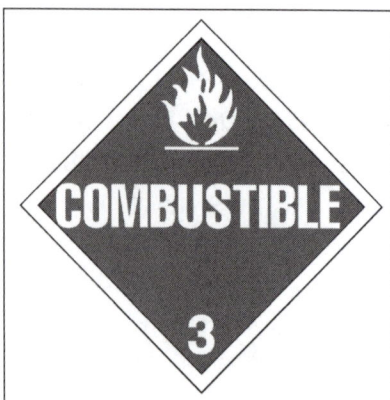

COMBUSTIBLE

3

Do not use supplemental oxygen while providing shocks from an AED. Turn off the oxygen or move it several feet away from the victim prior to providing a shock.

The use of an AED in a combustible environment where fumes or gases are present can be hazardous. If there is potential for ignition of combustible gases or fumes, such as oxygen or gasoline, do not use the AED until the hazardous atmosphere is eliminated or the victim is removed from the environment.

CONTROL OF BLEEDING

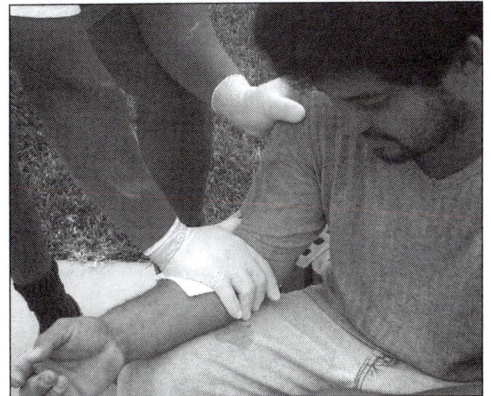

After completing the "ABCD" assessment, consider the "**S**" in ABCD'S: severe bleeding and shock.

Control bleeding with direct pressure. Apply firm pressure directly over the wound until the bleeding has stopped completely. This is the primary first aid treatment for bleeding.

Treat for shock by elevating legs and maintaining body temperature.

ELECTRICAL SHOCK

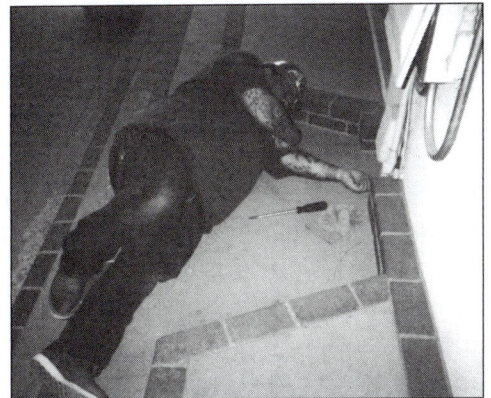

Electrical shock can cause breathing or circulation to suddenly stop. When dealing with an electrical shock, your own safety is the primary concern.

Before providing first aid, make sure:

- The patient is not touching the power source.
- The power source has been shut off.

All victims of electrical shock should be evaluated by a physician.

COLD TEMPERATURE

In a cold environment, the body's metabolism slows down, reducing the need for oxygen. As a result, brain cells take longer to die. Do not assume it is too late to start CPR. Breathing may be difficult to detect.

HYPOTHERMIA

If the victim is not breathing, begin CPR immediately. If the victim is responsive, gently remove him or her from the environment, remove damp clothing, dry and insulate. Keep the victim as still as possible, and activate EMS.

DROWNING

Remove the victim quickly from the water, but pay attention to your own safety. Begin CPR immediately.

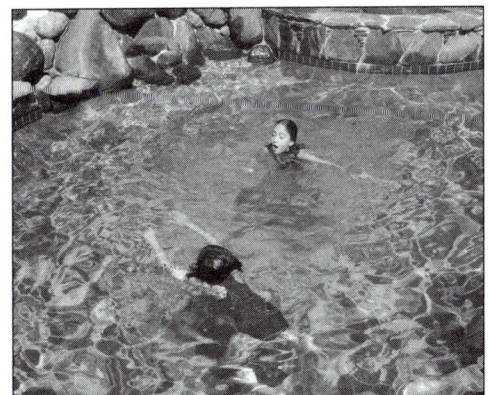

Make sure that nothing interferes with AED pad placement. This could block the flow of energy and prevent effective defibrillation.

AED USE ON CHILDREN (AGES 1 - 8)

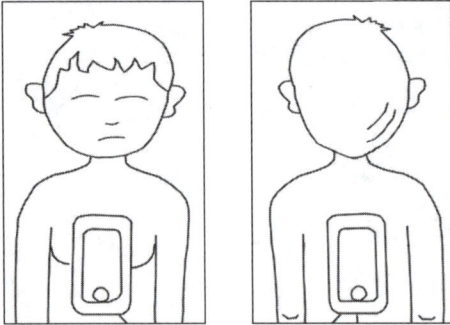

Change pad placement for a small child to 1 pad on front and 1 on back to avoid overlapping if needed.

Pediatric AED equipment adapts the waveform technology and reduces the amount of energy delivered. It is used on children older than one year and weighing less than 55 lbs. If a pediatric pad or adaptor is not available, adult AED equipment or pads can be used on a child.

- Do not use pediatric pads on an adult, because they will not deliver enough energy to defibrillate the adult heart.
- Do not overlap or cut pads.
- Follow AED manufacturer's recommendations for pad placement.

There is currently no recommendation for or against AED use on infants.

HAIRY CHEST

Chest hair that limits the contact between the electrodes and the skin can make it difficult for the AED to read the cardiac rhythm and deliver a shock. Use a razor to shave the chest in the area of electrode placement. If the electrodes have already been placed and the AED cannot analyze the heart rhythm, remove the pads with a quick movement to remove chest hair, and apply a new set of electrodes.

IMPLANTED DEVICES

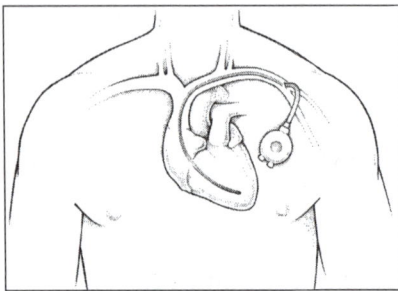

Some patients have electrical devices, such as a pacemaker or internal defibrillator, surgically implanted into their bodies. These will appear as a small, hard lump under the skin of the chest or abdomen. Do not place an electrode directly over an implanted device. Adjust the pad placement to at least 1 inch away from the device. If an internal defibrillator does deliver a shock (patient's muscles suddenly contract), wait 30 - 60 seconds to use the AED to avoid conflict between the two devices.

MEDICATION PATCHES

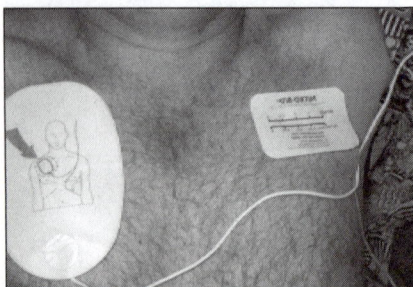

Medications can be embedded in an adhesive patch that is applied to the skin. Using the AED over a patch can burn the skin or block electrical impulses. Use a gloved hand to remove medication patches that interfere with pad placement. Wipe the skin clean with a towel before attaching the AED electrodes.

While working out at the local gym, you notice a man collapse. He doesn't appear to be moving, and no one seems sure what to do.

Place the action steps in correct sequence.

_____ Ask a bystander to call 911 and get the AED.

_____ Perform CPR for 2 minutes; use the AED as soon as it arrives.

_____ Assess responsiveness: Tap and Shout.

_____ Assess breathing for 5 – 10 seconds. Give 2 rescue breaths.

_____ Open the airway.

You are **alone** when you notice a child who appears to be unresponsive on the school playground.

Place the action steps in correct sequence.

_____ Go call 911 and get the AED.

_____ Perform CPR for 2 minutes.

_____ Assess responsiveness: Tap and Shout.

_____ Assess breathing for 5 – 10 seconds. Give 2 rescue breaths.

_____ Open the airway.

The technique to manage choking is the same for adults and children age 1 and older. Any time a person **suddenly** stops breathing, becomes cyanotic (blue), and eventually unresponsive, consider choking as a potential cause, especially in a younger victim.

Consider a victim's activities to help you recognize a choking emergency. Look for the **universal sign of choking** – one or both hands at the throat.

MILD OBSTRUCTION

With a mild airway obstruction, the victim is able to cough forcefully or even speak. If a victim can speak, he or she can breathe.

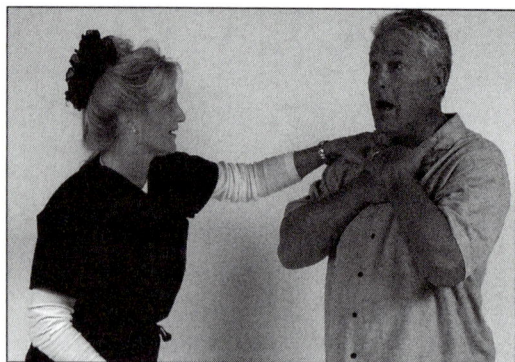

Mild obstruction – encourage cough

1. Observe for the universal sign of choking.
2. Ask the victim, "Are you choking?"
3. If the victim can cough forcefully or speak, do not interfere.
   a. Encourage him or her to cough.
   b. Observe for progression to severe obstruction.
4. If prolonged, send a bystander to call 911; do not leave the victim.

SEVERE OBSTRUCTION

A victim with a severe airway obstruction is unable to breathe, cough effectively, or speak. Immediate action is required to remove the obstruction, or the victim will soon become unresponsive and die.

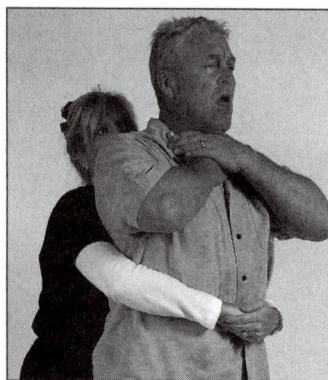

Severe obstruction – continuous abdominal thrusts

1. Observe for the universal sign of choking.
2. Ask the victim, "Are you choking?"
3. If the victim nods 'yes' or is unable to speak or cough:
   a. Send a bystander to call 911.
   b. Stand or kneel behind the patient and locate the navel with two fingers.
   c. Make a fist with your other hand and place it just above the navel. Grasp the fist with your free hand.
   d. Perform forceful inward and upward abdominal thrusts until the object is expelled or the patient becomes unresponsive.

CHEST THRUSTS - LARGE OR PREGNANT VICTIM

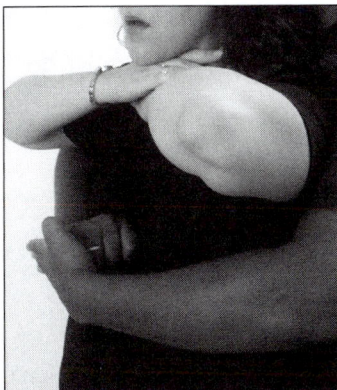

If a victim is pregnant or large, use **chest thrusts** instead of abdominal thrusts.

1. Stand behind the victim and reach around the chest, under the armpits.
2. Place one fist in the middle of the breastbone.
3. Grasp the fist with your other hand.
4. Perform continuous backward thrusts until the victim can breathe or becomes unresponsive.

UNRESPONSIVE CHOKING VICTIM

When a choking victim becomes unresponsive, relieve the obstruction using the steps of CPR.

1. Pull the victim close to your body and carefully lower to the ground.
2. Shout for help or send a bystander to call 911 and get the AED.
   a. If alone with an **adult** victim, call 911, return and begin CPR.
   b. If alone with a **child** victim, perform CPR for 2 minutes, then call 911.
3. Each time the airway is opened, look for the object. If seen, remove it.
4. If the object is removed, open the airway and check for breathing.
5. If no breathing, continue CPR.

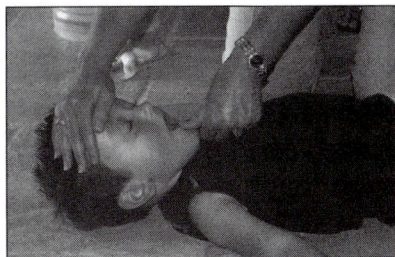

Check for Object

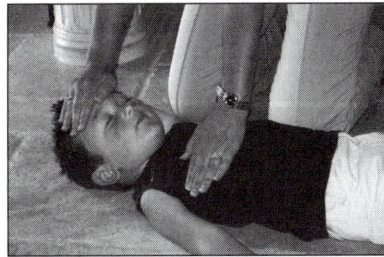

Perform CPR

CHOKING PREVENTION TIPS

1. Cut food into small pieces. Cut round food in half or quarters.
2. Chew food completely and eat slowly.
3. Do not talk or laugh with food in your mouth.
4. Avoid excessive alcohol intake.
5. Children should remain at the table while eating.
6. Protect infants and small children from objects that are small enough to fit through a household toilet paper roll.
7. Denture wearers should exercise extra care when eating.

Foods that commonly cause choking include meat, grapes, popcorn, peanut butter, round carrot slices, and hard candy.

Most episodes of choking in infants and young children occur when parents or caregivers are close by, usually during eating or play. Liquids such as juice or formula are the most common obstructions in infants.

An infant will not be able to give the universal sign of choking. Be alert and recognize the signs:

- Unable to cry or make sounds
- Weak, ineffective cough or cry
- Bulging, tearing eyes
- Difficult or absent breathing
- Blue or flushed face
- Panic or distressed facial expression

MILD OBSTRUCTION

1. Observe for signs of choking.
2. Determine if the infant can cough forcefully or breathe.
3. If the victim can cough or cry, do not interfere. Observe for complete obstruction.
4. If prolonged, send bystander to call 911; do not leave the infant.

SEVERE OBSTRUCTION

An infant with a severe airway obstruction is unable to make sounds, cry or cough.

1. Observe for signs of choking.
2. Determine if the infant can cough forcefully or breathe.
3. If the victim cannot cough or cry:
   a. Send a bystander to call 911, or carry the infant to the phone.
   b. Sit or kneel down and place the infant face down on your forearm with the head slightly lower than the chest. Rest your forearm on your thigh.
   c. Give 5 sharp back blows with the heel of your hand between the shoulder blades.
   d. Support the infant between your arms and turn face up, with the head lower than the chest.
   e. Give 5 chest thrusts (same location as chest compressions, but slower).
   f. Repeat the sequence of 5 back blows and 5 chest thrusts until the obstruction is removed or the victim becomes unresponsive.

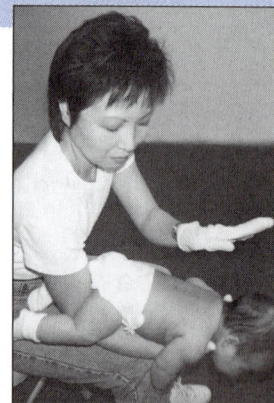

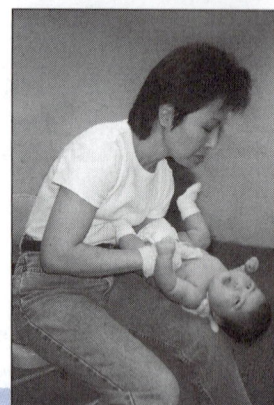

UNRESPONSIVE CHOKING VICTIM

When a choking victim becomes unresponsive, relieve the obstruction using CPR.

1. Place the infant on a firm, flat surface.
2. Shout for help or send a bystander to call 911.
3. Start CPR.
4. Each time the airway is opened, look for the object. If seen, remove it.
5. If the object is removed, open the airway and check for breathing.
6. If no breathing, continue CPR.
7. Call 911 after 2 minutes of CPR, then continue CPR.

ABCD'S	Adult (8 & older)	Child (1 - 8)	Infant (< 1)
Establish Responsiveness	Tap and shout	Tap and shout	Flick feet and shout
Activate EMS	Shout for help Send bystander	Shout for help Send bystander	Shout for help Send bystander
If alone:	Get help *before* ABCD'S	Get help *after* 2 minutes CPR	Get help *after* 2 minutes CPR Carry to phone
Open Airway	Head tilt/chin lift	Head tilt/chin lift	Head tilt/chin lift Neutral position
Check Breathing for 5-10 seconds If none, Give 2 Breaths	Pinch nose 1 second each Enough for chest rise	Pinch nose 1 second each Enough for chest rise	Into mouth and nose 1 second each Enough for chest rise
Chest Compressions:	**Press firm and fast.**	**Allow full chest recoil.**	**Decrease interruptions.**
Location	Center of chest between nipples	Center of chest between nipples	Center of chest just below nipple line
Technique	2 hands	1 or 2 hands	2 fingers
Compression Depth	$1\frac{1}{2}$ to 2 inches	$\frac{1}{3}$ to $\frac{1}{2}$ depth of the chest	$\frac{1}{3}$ to $\frac{1}{2}$ depth of the chest
Compression Rate	100/minute	100/minute	100/minute
Compression: Ventilation Ratio	30:2	30:2	30:2
Defibrillation	**Adult**	**Child**	**Infant**
Use AED	As soon as it arrives Adult pads	After 2 minutes CPR Ped pads/adaptor preferred	No recommendation
Choking	**Adult**	**Child**	**Infant**
Responsive Choking Victim	Continuous abdominal thrusts	Continuous abdominal thrusts	Continuous cycles of 5 back blows and 5 chest thrusts
Unresponsive Choking Victim	Perform Adult CPR Look in mouth before breaths Remove object if seen	Perform Child CPR Look in mouth before breaths Remove object if seen	Perform Infant CPR Look in mouth before breaths Remove object if seen

When assessing an emergency situation, use a systematic method to determine the seriousness of the emergency and what actions to take.

Activate EMS for any of the following:

- Difficulty breathing
- Chest pain or discomfort for 5 minutes
- Sudden weakness, slurred speech or severe headache
- Altered mental status or unresponsiveness
- Severe injury or illness
- Electric shock
- Seizure
- Any problem involving pregnancy
- Severe bleeding
- Critical burn
- Severe pain
- Suspected poisoning

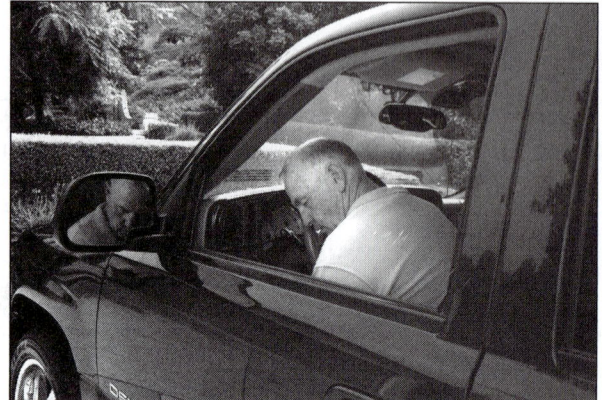

There are four phases of assessment:

1. **Scene Size-Up**
2. **Initial Assessment**
3. **Head-To-Toe Assessment**
4. **On-Going Assessment**

SCENE SIZE-UP

Quickly determine important information about an emergency scene.

1. Consider scene safety: the toxic or hazardous potential of the environment; the need for specialized rescue training, protection or equipment.
2. Determine the **mechanism of injury** or nature of the illness. If unsure, treat as an injury.
3. Identify the number of victims.
4. Activate EMS.

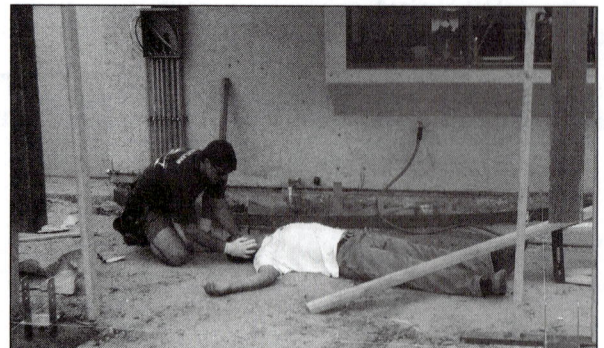

Do not move a victim; treat in the position found.

Only move a victim when the scene is unsafe, to open the airway, or begin CPR.

The **initial assessment** is used to establish responsiveness, identify and treat any life-threatening conditions, and determine the chief complaint.

1. **Establish Response:** Tap and shout at the patient. Assess the response:
   - Responsive and Aware
     ◆ Alert
     ◆ Able to answer simple questions
   - Altered Mental Status
     ◆ Confused
     ◆ Non-verbal (moaning or groaning)
     ◆ Abnormal behavior
   - Unresponsive

2. **Perform ABCD'S:**

   Unresponsive patient: Perform CPR if needed.

   Responsive patient:

   A – Is the **A**irway open?
   　　　If patient is able to speak, the airway is open.

   B – Is the patient **B**reathing normally?
   　　　• Abnormal breathing includes breathing too fast or slow, noisy or labored breathing, and speaking in short sentences.
   　　　• Flushed or bluish skin color may also indicate difficulty breathing.

   C – Are **C**ompressions needed?
   　　　A responsive patient does not need chest compressions.

   D – Is **D**efibrillation needed?
   　　　A responsive patient does not require defibrillation.

   S – Is there evidence of **S**evere bleeding or **S**hock?
   　　　• **Severe bleeding:** Look from head to toe for blood-soaked clothing, blood spurting from a wound, or signs of internal bleeding.
   　　　• **Shock:** Look and feel for pale, cool, moist skin.
   　　　　◆ Normal skin signs are warm, dry, and good color.
   　　　　◆ Victims with darker pigmentation may be checked at nail beds or on the inside of the lip.

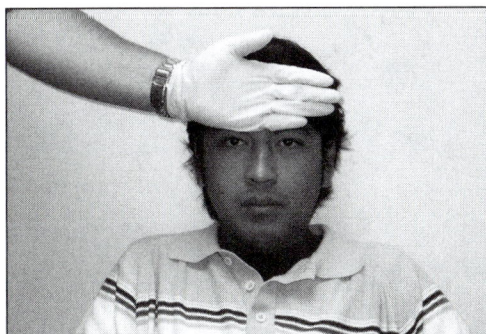

Place your forearm or the back of your hand against the patient's forehead.

Perform ABCD'S. Do not continue patient assessment until impairments in ABCD'S have been assessed and treated.

3. **Chief Complaint** (what is bothering the patient the most). Use the **PQRST** assessment to describe the chief complaint.

> **P:** What <u>P</u>rovoked the pain/problem? What makes it better or worse?

> **Q:** Describe the <u>Q</u>uality of the pain/problem (e.g. pressure, aching, numbness).

> **R:** What is the <u>R</u>egion of the pain/problem? Does it <u>R</u>adiate anywhere else?

> **S:** What is the <u>S</u>everity of the pain: mild, moderate or severe?

> **T:** How much <u>T</u>ime has passed since the episode began?

HEAD-TO-TOE ASSESSMENT

The head-to-toe assessment is a comprehensive, hands-on physical exam to check for injuries and other areas of discomfort. It should be performed in the position in which the patient is found. Observe for **signs** (what you see) and **symptoms** (what the patient tells you).

Gently palpate (feel) key areas and observe for pain (grimacing). Check for blood or other fluids on your gloved hands as you move from region to region.

Begin at the neck. *If the patient has neck pain/discomfort, immediately discontinue the assessment and stabilize the head and neck as a unit.* **Do not move the patient.**

Use the acronym **DOTS** to help focus your assessment:

> **D**: Deformities

> **O**: Open injuries

> **T**: Tenderness

> **S**: Swelling

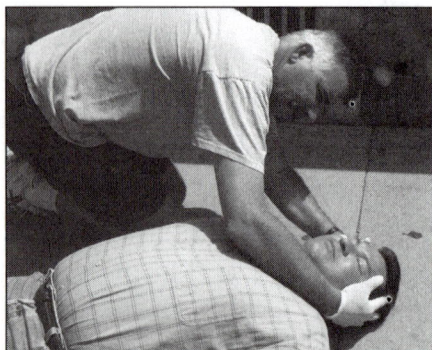 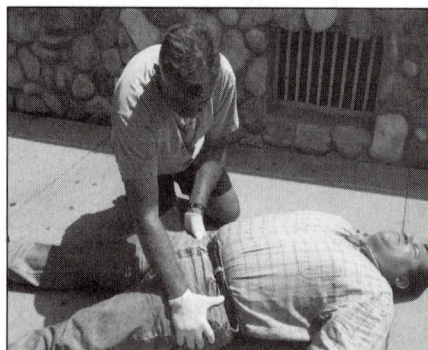 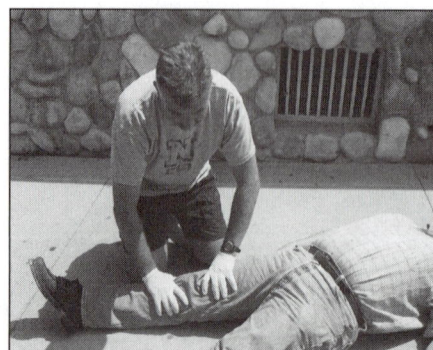

Head-To-Toe Assessment Sequence:

1. **Neck**: If the neck is painful or tender, stop the assessment and stabilize the head and neck as a unit in the position found.

2. **Head**: Eyes should move symmetrically; observe for drainage from the nose or ears, skull depressions, and blood or loose teeth in the mouth that may compromise the airway.

3. **Chest**: Discomfort, unequal rise and fall, difficulty breathing

4. **Abdomen**: Pain, bruising, rigidity, guarding

5. **Pelvis**: Pain, asymmetry

6. **Back**: Do not move the patient to check the back; if it is accessible, check for injuries.

7. **Extremities**: Range of motion, equal movement and normal sensation

On-Going Assessment

While waiting for EMS personnel to arrive, continue your assessment.

1. Ensure the scene is still safe.
2. Continually monitor the ABCD'S.
3. Observe for changes in mental status.

Establish a **medical history**. Use the acronym **SAMPLE** to remember what to ask.

S: What are the <u>S</u>ymptoms?

A: Are there any <u>A</u>llergies to medication?

M: Is the patient taking any <u>M</u>edication?

P: Is there any pertinent <u>P</u>ast History?

L: What was the patient's <u>L</u>ast <u>O</u>ral <u>I</u>ntake (liquid or solid, time, quantity)?

E: What <u>E</u>vents lead up to the injury or illness?

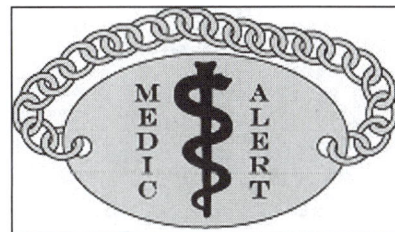

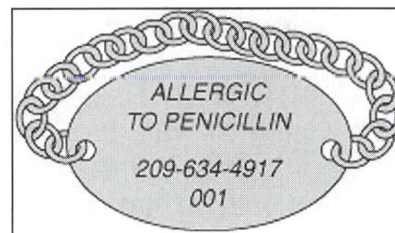

Check for medical alert tags.

DRAGS

Drags generally provide no cervical spine stabilization and should only be used when the rescuer and patient are in immediate danger and a rapid move is required.

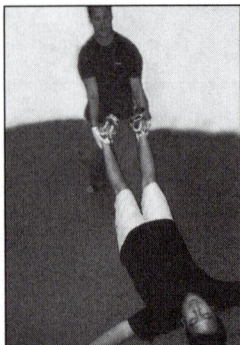

Ankle Drag: Grab the victim's ankles and drag to safety.

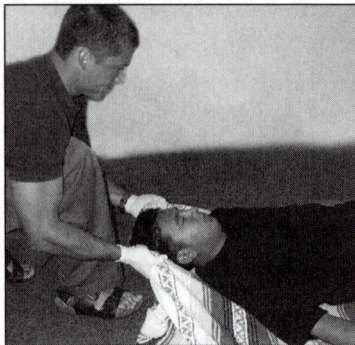

Blanket Drag: Place the victim on a blanket using the log roll technique. Support the head and neck with your forearms and drag to safety.

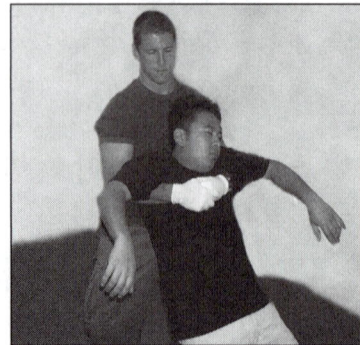

Shoulder Pull: Kneel down behind the victim's head and neck. Reach under armpits and interlace fingers. Support head and neck, stand with knees and drag to safety.

RESPONSIVE VICTIM CARRIES

Use only when the patient and rescuer's safety is compromised.

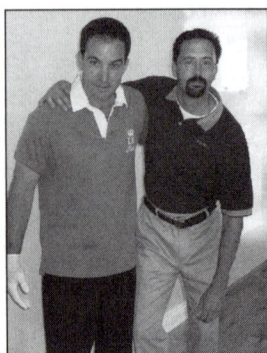

Human Crutch: Help the victim to walk by supporting the injured leg and helping him or her walk on the good leg.

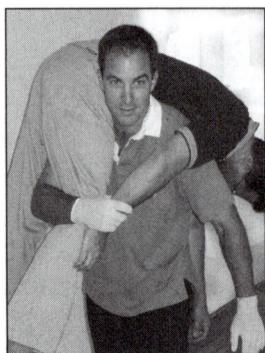

Fireman's Carry: Place the victim over your shoulder. This carry is good for lone rescuers who have to go long distances.

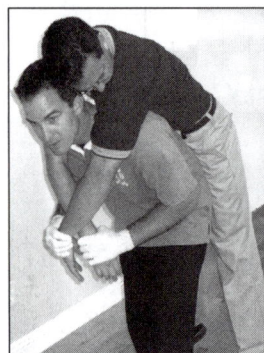

Pack-Strap Carry: This carry is good for moving injured patients long distances.

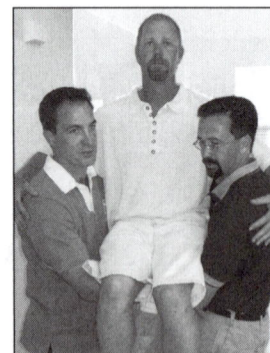

Seat Carry: Grasp hands or use the four-handed technique by inter-linking the rescuers' forearms and creating a 'seat.' The victim should hold on to the rescuers' shoulders.

Bleeding is the body's way of cleansing a wound. Many minor wounds will stop bleeding without intervention. The first responder is simply helping with the process. Severe, uncontrolled bleeding, however, is life threatening.

Direct pressure on the wound will control most bleeding. Apply direct pressure until the bleeding has stopped completely or professional rescuers arrive.

- **Arterial:** Bright red blood spurting from wound
- **Venous:** Dark red blood slowly flowing from wound
- **Capillary:** Blood slowly draining from wound

Arterial bleeding is the most serious due to the amount and speed of blood loss, and it is also the hardest type to control.

TYPES OF WOUNDS

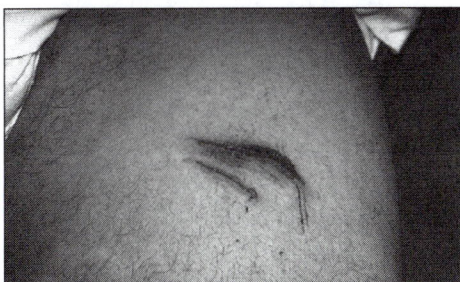

Laceration - Clean break of skin usually made with sharp object.

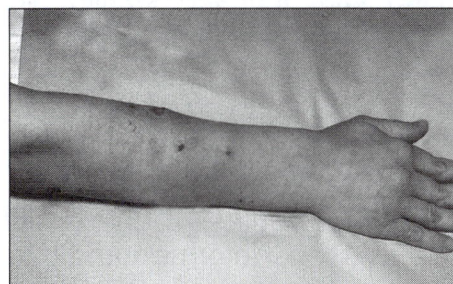

Puncture - Usually deep with minimal bleeding. Greatest chance of infection.

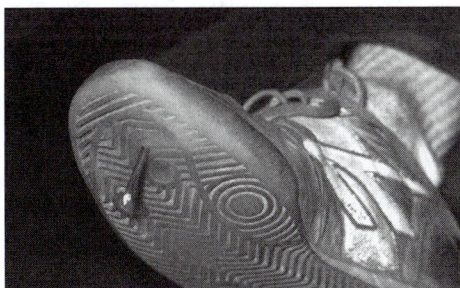

Impaled object - Foreign body penetration.
- Leave object in place, as it may slow bleeding.
- Use a bulky dressing and adhesive tape to stabilize object in place.

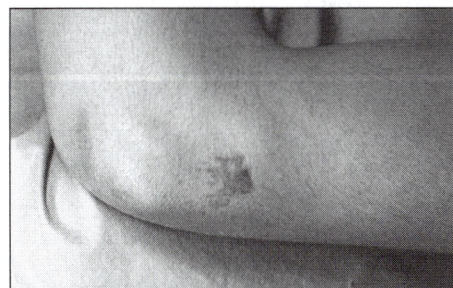

Abrasion - Painful scraping away of skin.

Amputation - Loss of body part.
- Apply pressure.
- Wrap amputated part in dry sterile gauze. Put gauze in plastic bag. Put plastic bag into second bag filled with ice. Do not let ice come in contact with part or immerse in water.

Avulsion - A piece of skin or other tissue is completely or partially torn from the body.
- Fold or replace torn skin if possible.
- Wrap the wound as a laceration.

SERIOUS WOUND TREATMENT:

1. Activate EMS and get the first aid kit.
2. Universal Precautions (gloves, mask, goggles, hand washing)
3. ABCD'S
4. Apply direct pressure.
5. Treat for shock - elevate legs and maintain body temperature.
6. Add dressings as they become soaked with blood; do not remove them.
7. Use an elastic or roller bandage to secure dressings in place and apply pressure.
8. Follow up with a physician.
9. Watch for signs of infection: redness, warmth, increased pain, drainage, swelling, fever.

MINOR WOUND TREATMENT:

1. Universal Precautions
2. Apply direct pressure.
3. Cleanse with soap and water. Irrigate for 5 minutes with clean tap water.
4. Apply a triple antibiotic ointment, if no allergy.
5. Cover with a sterile dressing.
6. See physician for tetanus shot.

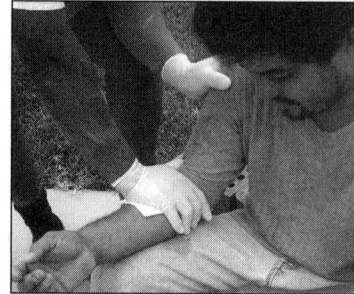

INTERNAL BLEEDING

Injury to internal organs can lead to bleeding that is concealed within the body and can be life-threatening. Swollen, deformed and painful extremities can also indicate internal bleeding.

SIGNS AND SYMPTOMS:

- Discolored, tender, swollen or hard skin or tissues, especially in abdominal area and suspected fracture sites
- Rapid respiratory and pulse rates
- Pale, cool, moist skin
- Abdominal pain, tenderness or rigidity
- Nausea, vomiting, coughing up blood
- Dark tarry or bright red stool
- Mental status change: confusion, irritability, unresponsiveness

TREATMENT:

1. ABCD'S
2. Activate EMS (call 911).
3. Calm and reassure the patient.
4. Treat for shock.
   - Position of comfort
   - Keep warm.
   - Elevate legs if indicated.
5. Monitor status.

NOSEBLEEDS

Nosebleeds are common and rarely life-threatening. The exception is a patient with a history of hypertension. This may be a warning sign of an impending stroke.

TREATMENT:

1. Sit patient in chair and lean slightly forward.
2. Pinch nostrils for several minutes.
3. Apply ice pack to bridge of nose if does not interfere with pressure.
4. DO NOT tilt head back or put head between knees.
5. Activate EMS if bleeding is very heavy, does not stop in 15 minutes, or difficulty breathing.

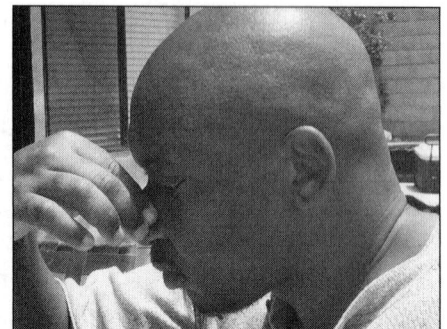

Shock is a life-threatening condition that occurs when there is inadequate blood flow to the vital organs and body tissues. Shock requires immediate medical treatment, or vital organs may fail. The goals of first aid care are to treat the underlying cause of shock, improve blood flow to the core of the body, and get medical help.

TYPES OF SHOCK

- **Hypovolemic:** Fluid or blood loss (bleeding, vomiting, diarrhea)
- **Cardiogenic:** Heart-related (heart attack)
- **Anaphylactic:** Allergic reaction (bee sting)
- **Neurogenic:** Nervous system injury
- **Septic:** Blood stream infection (blood poisoning)

SIGNS AND SYMPTOMS:

- Pale, cool, moist skin
- Weak, rapid pulse
- Rapid breathing
- Very low blood pressure (delayed capillary refill)
- Nausea or vomiting
- Emotional unrest or confusion
- Dizziness or faintness
- Unresponsiveness

TREATMENT:

1. ABCD'S
2. Activate EMS (call 911).
3. Lay the patient down and elevate feet about 12 inches.
4. Control external bleeding.
5. Maintain body temperature.
6. Monitor status every 5 minutes.
7. DO NOT give the patient anything to eat or drink.

Signs of shock are not always obvious. Suspect shock in cases of severe bleeding.

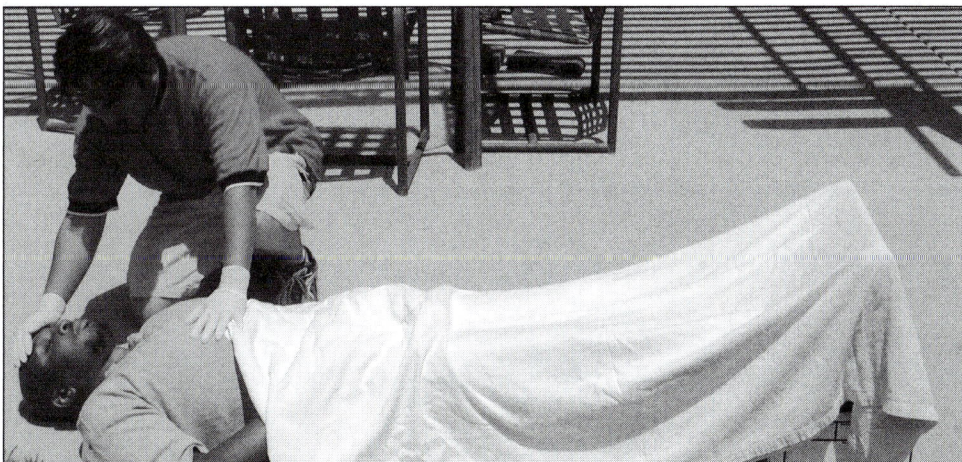

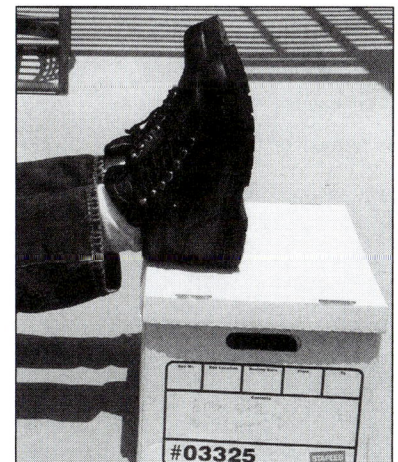

Do not elevate the legs in cases of neck, back, leg or head injury, heart attack or respiratory distress.

GUNSHOT WOUND (GSW)

The most important factor when dealing with gunshot wounds is scene safety. Once the scene is secure, turn your attention to patient care. Consider the following aspects of GSW:

- Causes laceration, crushing and shock wave-type injuries.
- May cause exit wounds that are larger and bleed more than entrance wounds.
- Can damage vital organs or major blood vessels.
- Can ricochet off bones, causing more damage.

TREATMENT:
1. Call 911 for EMS and law enforcement.
2. Ensure scene safety.
3. ABCD'S
4. Spinal immobilization if potential spinal injury.
5. Check for entrance and exit wound.
6. Control bleeding.
7. Keep patient still; treat for shock.
8. Do not disturb potential crime scene evidence.

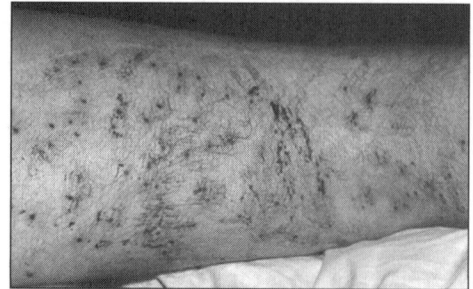
Example of shotgun wound

Gunshot victims usually require surgery to repair the damaged organs. Many GSWs are part of a crime; remember as much detail as you can and disturb as little of the crime scene as possible.

CRUSH INJURIES

Crush injuries occur when blunt force is applied to the body for extended periods of time (e.g. a car accident victim whose legs are trapped under the dashboard, or someone partially trapped under a heavy weight). The patient's outcome is determined by the length of time the tissue is compressed.

TREATMENT:
1. Scene safety
2. Activate EMS.
3. ABCD'S
4. Spinal immobilization
5. Treat soft tissue injuries.

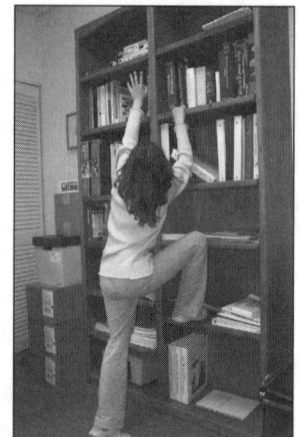

The primary concern is that the tissues are not being supplied with blood while under compression. Emergency scenes that involve crush injuries are typically dangerous; secondary collapse should be considered a major hazard.

IMPALED OBJECT

TREATMENT:
1. Leave the object in place, unless impaled in the cheek. Removing it may cause additional damage or increase bleeding.
2. ABCD'S
3. Activate EMS.
4. Expose the area; remove clothes, unless doing so may move the object.
5. Secure at least 3/4 of the object in place with bulky dressings or cloths to reduce movement.
6. Calm and reassure the patient.

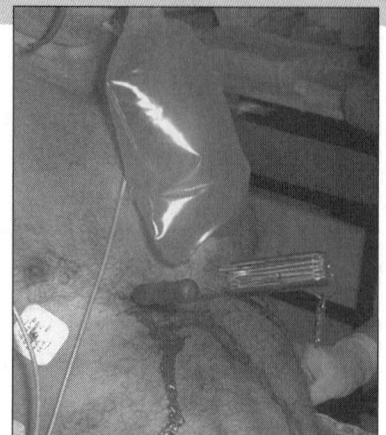

Head injuries can be external, involving the scalp, or internal, involving the skull, blood vessels or brain itself. Skull fractures may be obvious with open wounds, or assumed because of how the injury occurred or pain in the affected area. A **concussion** is a bruise to the brain, and is caused by a violent jolt or blow to the head. A serious brain injury can be life-threatening. All head injuries should be evaluated by a physician.

When caring for a victim with a potential head injury, perform the ABCD'S and treat the patient in the position found. Assume the patient also has a neck injury, and **stabilize the head and neck together to prevent further injury.** Do not continue the patient assessment.

SIGNS AND SYMPTOMS:

- Head trauma (bleeding, bruising, localized swelling, soft spots or indentations)
- Headache
- Raccoon's eyes (swelling and bruising under eyes)
- Bruising behind the ears
- Confusion, amnesia, repetitive questions
- Slurred speech
- Nausea and vomiting
- Difficulty with movement or sensation
- Blurred vision
- Unequal pupils
- Bleeding from nose, ears, eyes
- Seizures
- Unresponsiveness
- Ringing in the ears (tinnitus)

TREATMENT:

1. ABCD'S
2. Activate EMS (call 911).
3. Immobilize cervical spine (neck).
4. Control bleeding (do not apply direct pressure to a suspected skull fracture, as this may increase pressure to the skull).
5. Monitor mental status.
6. Apply an ice pack to the bruised area to control swelling. Do not apply pressure.

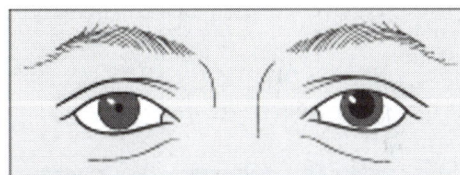

Unequal pupils

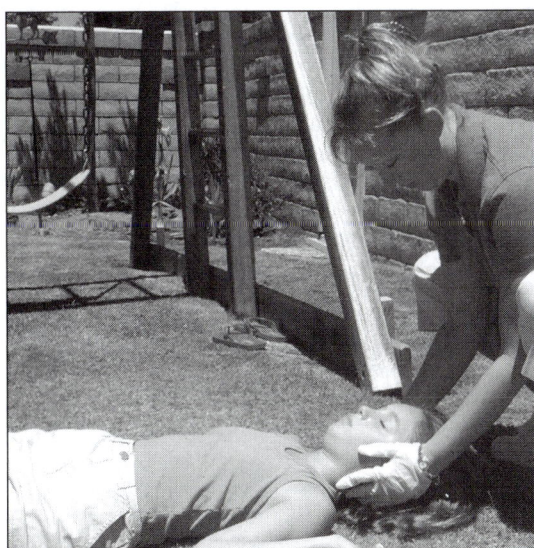

Deformity of the skull

Racoon's eyes

Fluid draining from the ears or nose

Battle's sign

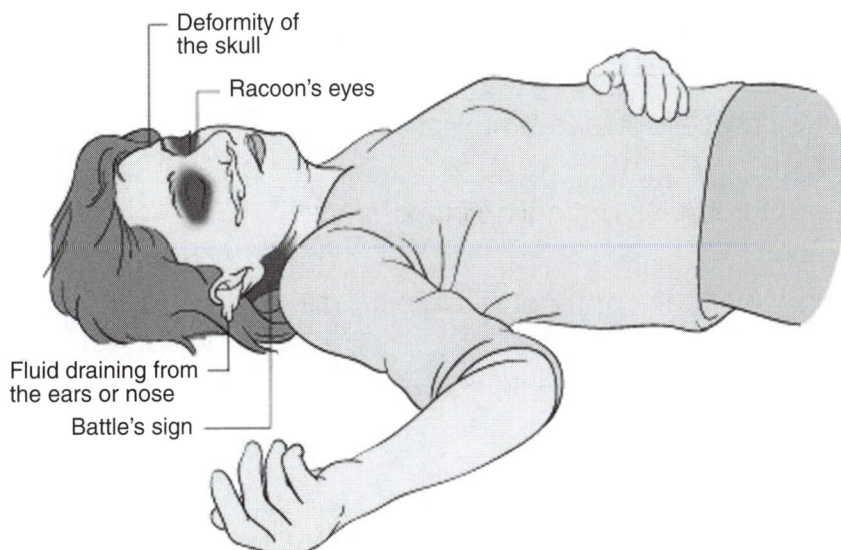

The spinal cord is a group of nerve tracts extending along the back, originating in the brain and ending in the spinal nerves that go to the various parts of the body. It is protected by the vertebral column, a series of bones (vertebrae) that extends from the base of the skull to the tailbone. When a traumatic event damages the cells within the spinal cord, it can result in loss of movement, sensation, and other activities such as breathing and bladder control.

Approximately 12,000 people suffer spinal cord injuries annually in the US; as many as 50% will die. The initial care of a victim with a spinal injury may affect the rest of his or her life. Proper handling is critical. High-risk incidents include motor vehicle accidents, severe blunt trauma, penetration injuries, diving injuries, head injuries, falls, lightning strikes, and any incident in which the victim is unresponsive for an unknown reason. If there is a chance of spinal injury, assume there is one.

Injury to the neck is especially devastating. The neck contains the airway, major blood vessels, and spinal cord tracts which innervate the respiratory muscles and all four limbs. If a victim has a head injury, assume there is also a neck injury.

DO NOT MOVE A VICTIM OF A SEVERE INJURY UNLESS:

1. You need to open or maintain an open airway, or perform CPR. If the patient vomits, carefully log roll him or her to the side, supporting the head, neck and back to prevent twisting.

2. There is imminent danger. Move the patient using a drag or pull; keep head and spine completely supported and aligned. Improper movement of an injured person can cause severe spinal cord injury.

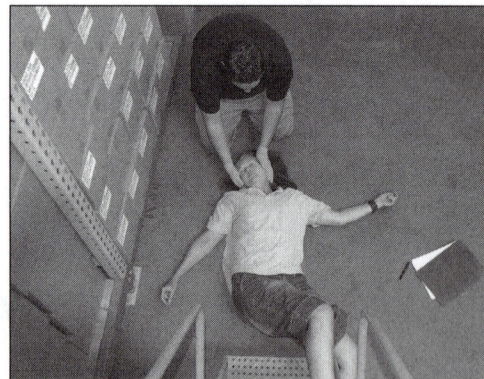

Immobilize in the position found.

SIGNS AND SYMPTOMS:	TREATMENT:
• Head, neck or back injury or pain	1. ABCD'S
	2. Maintain neck immobilization.
• Unresponsive trauma victim	a. Use the palms of your hands to support head in the position found.
• Numbness or tingling in extremities	b. Maintain an open airway with a head tilt/chin lift if needed.
• Weakness or paralysis in extremities	3. Activate EMS (call 911).
	4. Reassure patient; keep calm and still.
• Loss of bowel or bladder control	5. DO NOT move patient except for airway management or imminent danger.
	a. Move long axis (drag, pull)
• Difficulty breathing	b. Maintain neck immobilization.

KNOCKED-OUT PERMANENT TOOTH

Handle the tooth by the biting edge. Be careful not to touch the root. Rinse in water, but do not scrub it. Place the tooth in a container of cool milk. Have the patient bite down on a sterile gauze pad or clean cloth to control bleeding. Apply a cold pack to the face near the injury. **See a dentist within 30 minutes if possible** to replant the tooth. Watch for signs of airway compromise due to blood or broken teeth. Do not reinsert the tooth yourself.

TOOTHACHE

Although not a medical emergency, a toothache can be very painful. It is usually a sign of tooth decay, and is a common problem with a long onset. Field treatment options are limited, and include rinsing the mouth with water, and removing any food trapped between the teeth with dental floss. Do not medicate the tooth. Seek care from a dentist as soon as possible.

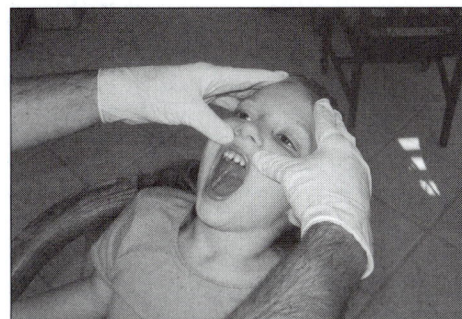
When assessing dental emergencies, keep fingers clear of the mouth.

JAW INJURY

To reduce pain from a possible jaw fracture, immobilize the jaw by splinting it with gauze. If a gauze roll is unavailable, use a towel, shirt or necktie to secure the jaw. Avoid interfering with the airway and do not over-tighten. Remain alert for airway complications. Seek professional medical attention.

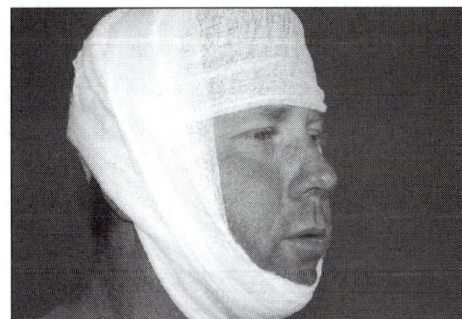

BITTEN/BLEEDING TONGUE OR LIP

Control bleeding by applying direct pressure to the affected area using a sterile gauze pad. Use ice wrapped in a cloth to keep swelling to a minimum. Apply continual pressure for at least six to ten minutes. If you are unable to control or stop the bleeding, activate EMS (call 911). Position the patient so that blood is allowed to drain out of the mouth, either sitting up with the head tilted slightly down, or in the recovery position. Observe for signs of airway compromise.

PENETRATING TRAUMA TO THE EYE

Penetrating trauma to the eye can be upsetting for the rescuer and the patient. Treatment of all penetrating traumas is directed at stabilizing the object, not removing it.

TREATMENT: PENETRATING EYE TRAUMA

1. ABCD'S
2. Calm the patient.
3. Send bystander to activate EMS.
4. Cover uninjured eye.
5. Use a cup, bulky dressing and gauze roll to stabilize the object in place.
   a. Remove the bottom of the cup, cutting a hole for the foreign object.
   b. Secure the foreign body with a sterile dressing.
   c. Place the hollow cup over the eye, being careful not to touch the foreign object.
   d. Secure the cup in place with gauze roll and tape.

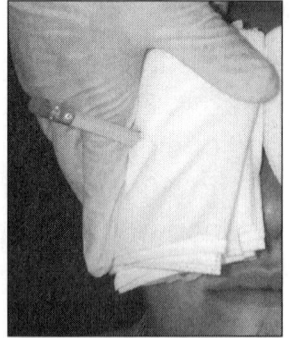

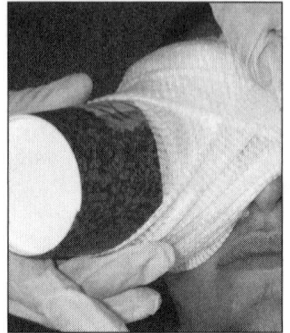

DEBRIS IN THE EYE

Small, loose foreign bodies in the eye will usually be removed by tears, which are natural flushing agents.

TREATMENT: DEBRIS IN THE EYE

1. Instruct victim to blink several times.
2. Gently flush the area with lukewarm water.
3. If flushing does not remove the object, use a swab or similar thin, stiff object and lay it across the top of the eyelid.
4. Fold the lid over the swab and flush the eye with lukewarm water, or attempt to remove with wet sterile gauze.
5. If you are unable to remove the source of irritation, seek medical care.
6. DO NOT rub the eye.

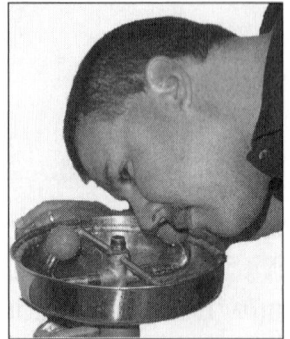

Chemical Injury

Tilt head down toward the affected eye, and apply a gentle stream of water to the bridge of the nose. Keep the affected eye lower than the unaffected eye. Flush the eye for at least 20 minutes. Remove contact lenses. Seek medical care immediately.

Corneal Abrasions

When the cornea (single layer of cells over the surface of the eye) becomes abraded, it is often described as a continual feeling that something is in the eye. A corneal abrasion must be evaluated by a physician.

Blow to the Eye

Gently apply a cold pack to reduce pain and swelling. Do not apply pressure to the eye. If the victim develops a black eye or changes in vision, see a physician immediately.

Rib Fracture or Flail Chest

Rib Fractures are painful but rarely life-threatening. Sharp bone ends can cause serious injuries such as a punctured lung or lacerated liver. Observe for signs of internal bleeding or respiratory distress; decrease patient movement.

A **Flail Chest** occurs when three or more ribs are broken in two or more places. Due to the instability of the chest wall, these broken ribs no longer function to aid in the process of breathing.

Signs and Symptoms:
- Consider how the injury occurred.
- Bruising
- Pain with a deep breath
- Tenderness
- Deformity
- Paradoxical movement: the flail segment moves in the opposite direction of the rest of the chest.

Treatment:
1. ABCD'S
2. Activate EMS.
3. Consider neck injury.
4. Place 2" wide adhesive tape over the flail section to "bond" the chest cavity, enabling it to function as a unit.

Sucking Chest Wound

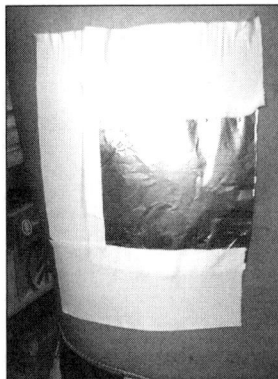

Three-sided dressing

Treatment:
1. ABCD'S
2. Activate EMS.
3. Keep patient still.
4. Apply airtight dressing (e.g. foil, plastic wrap, folded universal dressing) to keep air from entering during inhalation. Tape only three sides so air can escape during exhalation.

Trauma that has punctured the chest wall may create a sucking chest wound, a life-threatening condition. When the patient breathes, a sucking sound is produced by the passage of air through the wound. Air rushes into the chest cavity, collapsing the lungs.

Abdominal Wounds

An **open abdominal wound** is usually caused by a penetrating injury and may expose internal organs. In extreme cases, organs may protrude through the wound (evisceration). Do not attempt to replace abdominal organs or remove objects impaled in the abdomen.

A **closed abdominal wound** is usually caused by blunt trauma injury. Consider how the injury occurred and the need for neck immobilization. Common causes of internal bleeding are automobile accidents, knife and gunshot wounds, as well as medical problems related to the stomach and intestines.

All **pregnancy-related** abdominal injuries should be evaluated by a physician. Activate EMS at any sign of sudden illness, complication, or injury. Position a pregnant patient on her LEFT side.

Signs and Symptoms:
- Weak, rapid pulse
- Pale, cool, moist skin
- Abdominal pain, tenderness or rigidity
- Nausea or vomiting
- Dark tarry or bright red stools

Treatment:
1. ABCD'S
2. Activate EMS.
3. Position on back with knees bent if does not increase pain.
4. Treat for shock.
5. Stabilize foreign object with a bulky dressing. DO NOT REMOVE.
6. Cover eviscerated organs with a moist sterile dressing.
7. Do not give food or drink.

The human body is made up of more than 600 muscles and 200 bones. Muscles are firmly attached to bones through **tendons**, and provide active movement of the skeleton. A **joint** is the junction where two or more bones meet, and is supported by **ligaments**, muscles and a **joint capsule**.

FRACTURES AND DISLOCATIONS

A **fracture** is a break in a bone produced by excessive strain or force on the bone. Causes include a blow, a fall, a twisting movement, or even no apparent cause. An **open fracture** (compound) has penetration of skin and bleeding, while a **closed fracture** (simple) has the skin intact. A **dislocation** is a separation or displacement of joint surfaces. It is usually caused by an injury such as a hard blow or fall.

SIGNS AND SYMPTOMS:

- Swelling
- Bruising
- Deformity
- Pain
- Bleeding
- Inability to use the injured part
- Exposed bone ends (open fracture)
- Crackling sound with movement
- Numbness

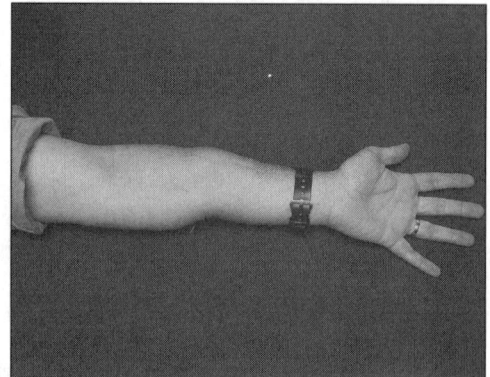

Remove rings and watches before splinting in case of swelling.

TREATMENT:

1. ABCD'S
2. Activate EMS.
3. Watch for signs of shock.
4. Cover open wounds with a sterile dressing; apply gentle pressure to control bleeding.
5. Stabilize and support the injury in the position found. Only splint the injury if emergency response is delayed or if you are far from medical care.
6. Monitor circulation and sensation beyond the injury site (numbness or tingling).
7. Apply a cold pack (20 minutes on, 20 minutes off) to reduce pain, swelling and bleeding.
8. DO NOT try to move a victim with a suspected fracture unless it is absolutely necessary.
9. DO NOT try to realign a broken bone or reduce a dislocation yourself.
10. DO NOT give the victim food or fluids. This may delay any necessary surgery.

Splinting is used for fractures, dislocations and severe sprains. **Applying a splint** reduces the movement of injured muscles and bones, and allows the patient to be transported with less pain and risk of further injury.

A splint can be made from a variety of rigid or firm materials, such as cardboard, a tree branch, a broom handle, or a tightly rolled blanket or magazine. An injured limb can also be protected by "buddy taping" it to another part of the body. **A splint should immobilize the areas above and below an injury, and should not cause increased pain.**

PROCEDURE:

1. Explain the procedure to the patient.
2. Select an appropriate splint. Make sure the splint is longer than the bone it will support.
3. Pad the splint with soft material to relieve local pressure and ensure even contact.
4. Carefully apply the splint. DO NOT straighten or manipulate the limb; splint in the position found.
5. Use tape or binding to secure the splint. It should be snug, but not so tight that it restricts blood flow.
6. Check sensation and capillary refill before and after splinting.

The splinting methods below are for short-term, emergency use. Only apply a splint to immobilize an injury during transport to seek medical care.

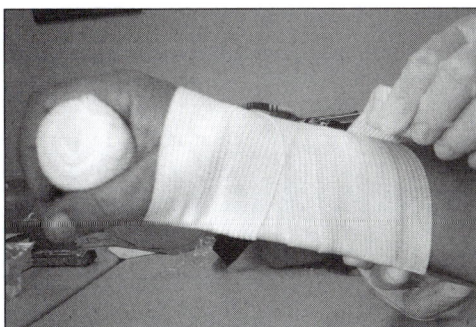

Wrist splint

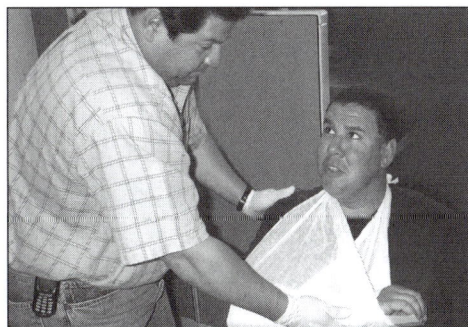

Arm in sling

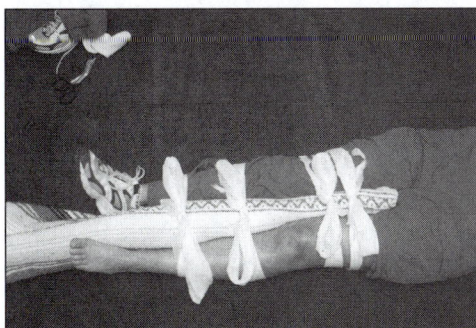

Leg splint

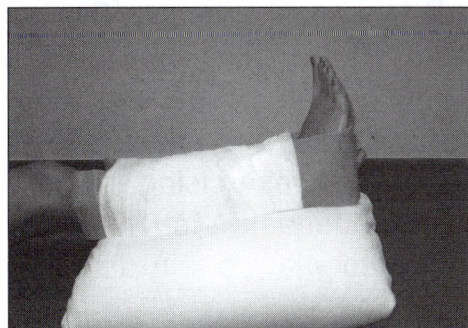

Ankle splint

SPRAINS, STRAINS AND CONTUSIONS

A **contusion** is bruising from a direct blow. A **sprain** is a tearing of ligaments or other structures in a joint, while a **strain** is a stretching or tearing of muscle or tendon (a pulled muscle). A sprain or strain occurs when a structure is stretched beyond its normal range of motion. If a sprain remains swollen and painful for several days, consult a physician. Fractures can often only be detected by x-ray.

Treat sprains, strains and contusions with the **RICE** technique:

REST	Stop activity after an injury. Do not move or put weight on the injured area.
IMMOBILIZE	Stablilize and support the injured area in the position found. Only apply a splint if the patient must be moved, and if it does not increase pain.
COLD	Apply an icepack wrapped in a thin cloth to reduce swelling, bleeding and pain. Apply the ice 20 minutes on, 20 minutes off. DO NOT apply ice directly onto the skin.
ELEVATE	Raise the injury above the heart to minimize swelling, if it does not increase the pain.

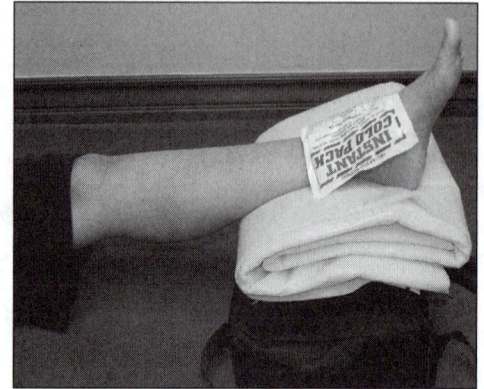

Tip: Avoid injury by warming up before exercise, and keeping your muscles and joints flexible with regular stretching.

MUSCLE CRAMPS

A muscle cramp occurs when a muscle is locked into an involuntary contraction or spasm lasting from a few seconds to several minutes. Symptoms can range from muscle twitching to severe pain with a hard bulging muscle. The exact cause is unknown, but it can involve muscle fatigue, overexertion, dehydration, exercising in extreme heat, pregnancy, or inadequate stretching. They may also be associated with certain diseases or medications.

TREATMENT:

1. Stop the activity that triggered the cramp.

2. Gently stretch the muscle until the spasm relaxes and the pain subsides.

3. Apply ice to the muscle to relax it.

Fast, effective burn treatment can reduce the degree of injury and even save a life. The young and the elderly have the most difficulty recovering from severe burns. Critical burn areas include:

- HEAD
- NECK
- HANDS
- FEET
- GENITALS

The preferred treatment for small or minor thermal burns is cooling the area with water. Cool water provides pain relief and will help stop the spread of the burn. If the victim begins to shiver, discontinue the cooling process. Remove any clothing or jewelry that does not stick to the burned skin. Jewelry retains heat and will continue to burn even after the heat source has been removed.

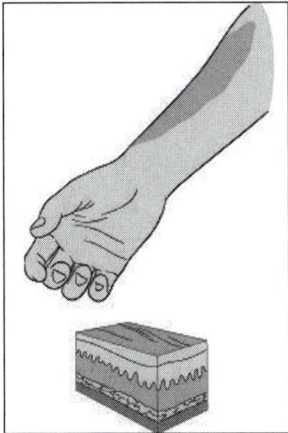

1st degree burn: burns the outer layer of skin (redness, pain, swelling)

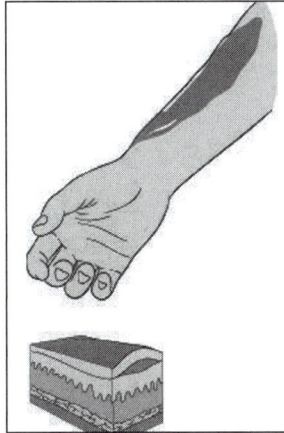

2nd degree burn: burns the second layer of skin (blisters, pain, swelling, red and splotchy appearance)

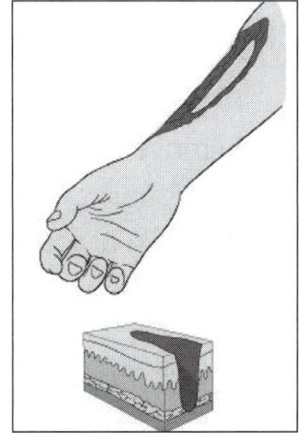

3rd degree burn: burns all layers of the skin and possibly more (no pain, may appear charred black or dry and white)

THERMAL BURNS

Thermal burns are caused by direct or radiant heat exposures to extreme temperatures. They result from fire, steam, or other exposure to increased temperature.

CHEMICAL BURNS

Large amounts of water are required to flush chemicals from the skin. Powdered chemicals should first be brushed from the skin, followed by flushing with water for 20 minutes. Ensure run-off water does not flow over unaffected skin or onto rescuer.

ELECTRICAL BURNS

The most important consideration when treating a victim with an electrical burn is to ensure scene safety. Do not touch the victim until the power has been turned off at the source. Once you are certain the power supply has been turned off, treat the burn. Electricity follows the path of least resistance through the body. Commonly there is an entrance and exit wound. **All victims of electrical burns need to be evaluated by a physician.**

BURN TREATMENT:

1. Ensure scene safety. If electrical burn is suspected, ensure power source is eliminated.
2. Extinguish flames (stop, drop and roll); remove victim from environment.
3. Activate EMS for a critical burn.
4. ABCD'S. Assess airway for evidence of respiratory tract burns such as singed hairs or soot around the mouth or nose.
5. Cool small or minor thermal burns with water until pain decreases.
6. Cover burn area with a dry, sterile dressing, or a clean sheet for large burn area. Keep as clean as possible to reduce risk of infection.
7. Assess for other life-threatening traumatic injuries.
8. Treat for shock.
9. Remove clothing or jewelry that does not stick.
10. Stop cooling process if patient begins to shiver.
11. Maintain an open airway and continue to monitor breathing.
12. DO NOT break blisters.
13. DO NOT apply ice directly to the skin.
14. DO NOT apply butter, ointment or creams to a severe burn.

ACTIVATE EMS FOR A CRITICAL BURN:

*   Burn to head, neck, hands, feet, or genitals
*   Large burn area or multiple burn sites
*   Burn to the airway or difficulty breathing. Airway burns cause swelling which may close the airway.
*   3rd degree burn to the elderly or very young
*   Chemical or electrical burn
*   Burn with other traumatic injuries

FIRE SAFETY TIPS:

1. If your clothes catch on fire, don't panic: stop, drop and roll.
2. Escape first, then call for help.
3. Know two ways to escape from every room.
4. Practice escape routes, and keep them free of clutter.
5. Do not open doors that are hot to the touch.
6. When escaping, never stand up; crawl low, and keep mouth covered.
7. Place smoke alarms in each room; change batteries annually.
8. Equip security bars or windows with a quick-release.

You are in a restaurant and observe a man clutching his throat. He is not making any sounds.

Place the action steps in correct sequence.

_____ Stand behind the victim.

_____ Place 1 fist just above his navel, and your other hand on top of your fist.

_____ Ask the victim, "Are you choking?"

_____ Perform abdominal thrusts until the food is expelled or the man becomes unresponsive.

_____ State that you are going to help.

You are working in a warehouse and notice a coworker lying at the bottom of the stairs, calling for help.

Place the action steps in correct sequence.

_____ Perform the Scene Size-up to determine if the scene is safe.

_____ Check the victim from head to toe for specific areas of injury.

_____ Perform the Initial Assessment to determine **responsiveness**, identify **life-threatening conditions** and **chief complaint**. Activate EMS if needed.

_____ Perform the On-going Assessment.

Acute (sudden) shortness of breath, a symptom of **respiratory distress**, is a medical emergency. There can be many causes, including injury, electrocution, heart attack, asthma, congestive heart failure (CHF), poisoning, allergic reaction, choking, emphysema, and bronchitis. Generally, the treatment for respiratory emergencies is the same. Fast recognition of the emergency and prompt activation of EMS (911) is critical. Delay can be fatal.

SIGNS AND SYMPTOMS:

Breathing rate: Too fast or too slow, agonal breathing (only a few breaths per minute)

Noisy breathing: Wheezing, gurgling, high-pitched whistle-like sound

Sitting upright: "Tripod" positioning

Labored breathing: Using shoulder and back muscles to assist breathing

Broken dialogue: Speaking in short sentences or one word answers, pausing for breath

Color: Ashen, pale, cyanotic (blue skin, lips, fingernail beds)

Children: Nasal flaring, rib retraction (movement of the ribs with breathing)

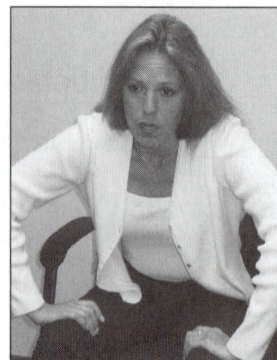

Tripod Position

ASTHMA

Asthma is a chronic disease in which the main air passages of the lungs become inflamed. During an asthma attack, the muscles around the airways tighten and extra mucus is produced. This results in narrowing of the airways and less air flow to the lungs.

Triggers that can cause or worsen an asthma attack include the following:

- Strong odors
- Exercise
- Emotional stress
- Respiratory infection
- Change in the weather
- Inhaled substances
- Irritants (e.g. dust, smoke, pollution)
- Allergens (e.g. pollen, pet dander)

An episode can occur with little warning. Recognize the symptoms and respond quickly.

SIGNS AND SYMPTOMS:
- Labored, rapid breathing
- Coughing
- Wheezing
- Shortness of breath
- Chest tightness
- Anxiety
- Upright, rigid posture
- Cyanosis
- Flared nostrils
- History of asthma

Early activation of 911 saves lives!

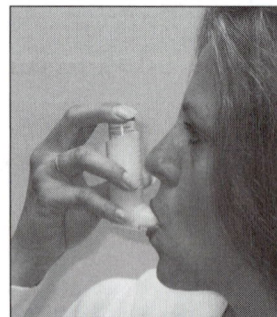

Many asthmatics carry inhaled bronchodilators that open narrowed air passages and ease breathing.

Call 911 immediately if you suspect a severe asthma attack or if an inhaled treatment isn't working.

Note: Check with your State EMS and workplace for requirements and guidelines on the use of inhaled medications.

TREATMENT:
1. ABCD'S
2. Help patient use inhaler if needed.
3. Determine attack trigger.
4. Call 911 if no relief from inhaler.
5. Position of comfort, usually sitting up.
6. Calm patient.

An **allergy** is an overreaction of your body's immune system to a substance (allergen). Approximately 50 million Americans suffer from allergies. When a person comes in contact with an allergen, the body releases a massive amount of **histamine**, a chemical which causes allergic symptoms. **The quicker the onset of symptoms, the more severe the reaction.**

The result can be **anaphylactic shock**, a severe allergic reaction which causes swelling in the airway and a sudden drop in blood pressure. Patients should never self-administer antibiotics prescribed for a friend or family member due to possible allergic reactions.

Common allergens:

- pollen
- bee sting venom
- shellfish
- dairy products

- drugs
- eggs
- chocolate
- nuts

Allergic reactions tend to get worse with each subsequent occurrence. People with known allergies may carry a self-injectable epinephrine kit to combat the allergic reaction.

Be sure to check for medical alert tags.

SIGNS AND SYMPTOMS:

- Hives, rashes, itchy skin
- Swollen face, eyes, throat, tongue
- Difficulty breathing, coughing, congestion
- Sneezing
- Tightness in the chest and throat
- Dizziness, confusion, agitation

TREATMENT:

1. ABCD'S
2. Activate EMS system.
3. If requested, help with auto injector, if you are trained and your state and workplace allow it.
4. Reassure patient.
5. If allergic reaction is due to a bee sting, quickly scrape off the stinger with a straight edged object.

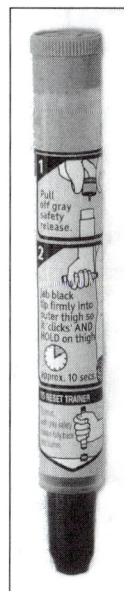

The EpiPen® is an example of an epinephrine auto injector.

Note: Check with your State EMS and workplace for requirements and guidelines for the use of an epinephrine auto injector.

USING AN EPINEPHRINE AUTO INJECTOR:

1. Remove the safety cap. Handle carefully.
2. Press the black tip firmly against the thigh.
3. Hold for 10 seconds.
4. Rub the injection site.
5. Follow sharps disposal procedure or give to EMS.

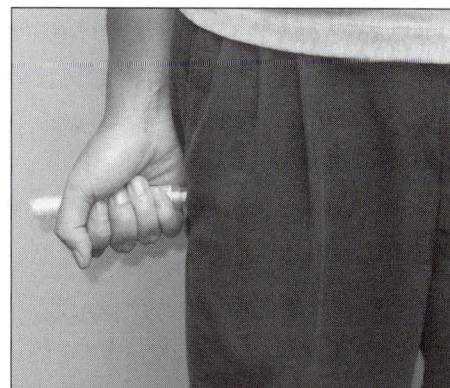

A **seizure** is an abnormal electrical discharge in the brain. The symptoms displayed will depend on the cause of the seizure and the part of the brain that is affected. It may affect only one part of the body (focal seizure), or may affect the whole body (generalized seizure). The most common cause of seizure is **epilepsy**. Other causes include brain tumor, brain injury, stroke, drug overdose, poisoning, low blood sugar, infection, or a sudden lack of oxygen to the brain. A seizure may last just a few seconds or several minutes. A physician should determine the cause of first time or repeated seizures.

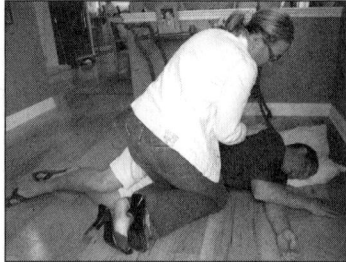

SIGNS AND SYMPTOMS:

- Muscle twitches, rigidity, violent rhythmic contractions
- Staring, eye movements, lip smacking, mouth movements, drooling, head turning, purposeless movements
- Abnormal sensations, hallucinations
- Nausea, sweating, dilated pupils, flushed skin, incontinence
- May become unresponsive or unaware of surroundings

TREATMENT DURING THE SEIZURE:
1. ABCD'S
2. Place patient on the floor; remove nearby objects.
3. Protect the victim's head from injury with a small pillow or other soft object.
4. Activate EMS (call 911).
5. Ask spectators to leave.
6. DO NOT put anything in victim's mouth.
7. DO NOT restrain victim.

TREATMENT AFTER THE SEIZURE:
1. Reassess ABCD'S.
2. If potential spinal injury, immobilize head and neck together to prevent further injury.
3. Place in recovery position.
4. Cool febrile seizure patient.
5. Ensure 911 has been called.

Febrile seizures are triggered by a rapidly increasing body temperature. They are most common during the first two years of life, but can be seen in children up to age four or five. If a febrile seizure is suspected, follow seizure treatment guidelines and begin to cool the febrile child with a cool, moist towel. Stop the cooling process if shivering or goose bumps appear.

FAINTING

Fainting is a brief period of unresponsiveness usually caused by a momentary lack of blood supply to the brain. It can be caused by dehydration, temporary low blood pressure or low blood sugar, or may be related to environmental, emotional or physical stress. Since fainting may also be related to a heart or other medical condition, contact your physician for evaluation. If you feel dizzy or faint, lie down.

SIGNS AND SYMPTOMS:

- Lightheadedness, disorientation
- Nausea
- Flushed, warm appearance
- Unresponsiveness

TREATMENT:
1. Use recovery or shock position until dizziness passes.
2. Loosen restrictive clothing.
3. Activate EMS if victim remains unresponsive or is injured.

Diabetes is a disease that decreases a person's ability to process sugar. Most of the food we eat is broken down into glucose, the form of sugar in the blood. Our bodies produce insulin to aid the movement of sugar from our blood into our cells to be used for energy. In people with diabetes, either little or no insulin is produced, or their cells do not respond appropriately to the insulin that is produced.

Millions of people have diabetes and live normal lives. While some can control it by proper diet, others need to take medication to keep it under control. High blood sugar is a problem that develops over several days. **Excessively low blood sugar is a life-threatening emergency that can develop in minutes.** It occurs when an individual has taken insulin but has not eaten, resulting in a sudden reduction of blood sugar.

SIGNS AND SYMPTOMS OF LOW BLOOD SUGAR:

- Altered mental status
- Pale, cool, moist skin
- Dizziness or headache
- Full, rapid pulse
- Rapid onset
- Tremor or seizures
- Double vision
- Weakness

TREATMENT:

1. ABCD'S
2. Activate EMS (call 911).
3. Position of comfort
4. If patient is responsive, give sugar (orange juice, cake frosting, honey, syrup, or a sugar and water solution).
5. If patient is drooling, he or she is unable to protect the airway; do not give food or drink.

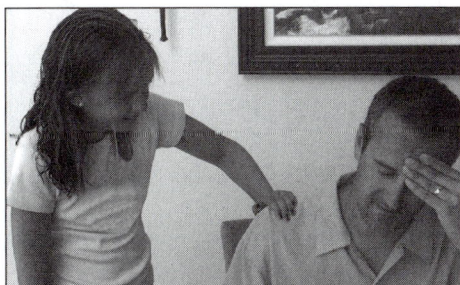

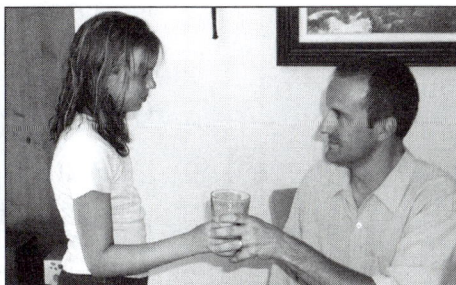

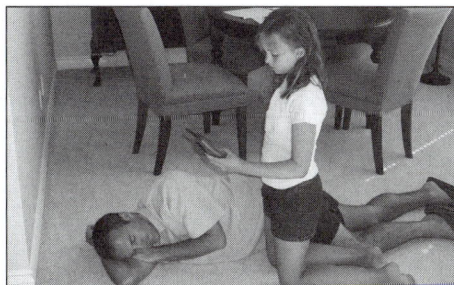

Note: Sugar administration is recommended in all diabetic emergencies. Untreated low blood sugar may cause serious brain damage. There is little risk of worsening the condition of a patient with high blood sugar.

A poison is any substance (solid, liquid or gas) that causes injury or death when it enters the body. More than 50% of poisonings occur in children younger than 6 years old. Approximately 90% of all poisonings occur at a residence.

Poisons enter the body in four ways:

- Ingestion: swallowing the poison

- Inhalation: breathing dust, gases, fumes or mists

- Absorption: through the skin

- Injection: hypodermic needle, bite or sting

POISONS ACT FAST – SO MUST YOU!

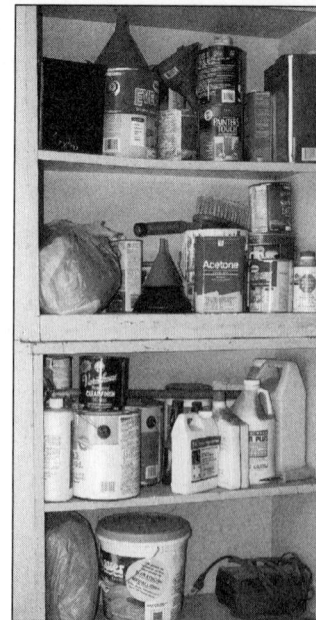

SIGNS AND SYMPTOMS:

- Throat pain; abdominal pain

- Nausea and vomiting

- Drooling or unusual odor on breath

- Altered level of response; behavior changes

- Sweating

- Diarrhea

- Difficulty breathing

- Seizures

- Burns, redness or blisters around the mouth

- Empty bottles or containers; disturbed plants

TREATMENT:

1. Check for scene safety and clues.

2. Remove victim if necessary.

3. ABCD'S

4. Place in a position of comfort.

5. Identify the poison, how much and when it was taken.

6. Contact EMS for a victim who is unresponsive or in distress.

7. Contact the Poison Control Center for a responsive victim in no distress.

8. Continue to monitor ABCD'S.

9. DO NOT give the victim food or drink unless instructed to do so.

POISON CONTROL CENTER

While waiting for EMS personnel to arrive, contact the Poison Control Center. They can advise you on the preferred treatment. **Never induce vomiting unless instructed to do so by a Poison Control Center or medical professional.**

In most regions, the Poison Control Center number is (800) 222-1222. Check the front of your phone book to find the Poison Control Center number in your area.

Swallowed Poisons

Commonly ingested poisons include household cleaning products, plants, chemicals, cosmetics, an overdose of medication or illegal drugs.

Since most poisonings involve children, it's important to child proof your home:

- Lock dangerous items out of sight and reach.
- Keep products in their original containers.
- Buy household products and medicines in child-resistant packages.
- Return products to safe storage immediately after use.
- Never call medicine "candy."
- Keep important phone numbers by every phone (e.g. EMS, Poison Control Center, police and fire departments, your physician).

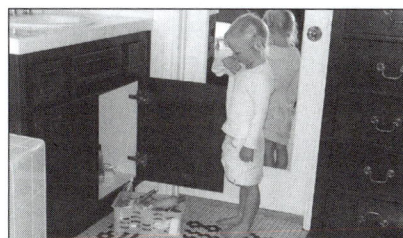

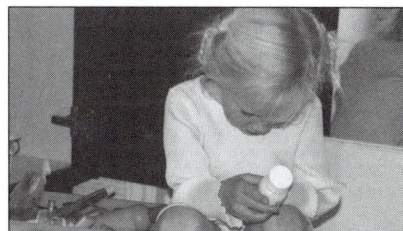

Inhaled Poisons

Inhalation hazards include pesticides, fumigants, smoke from fires, as well as chemical fumes, vapors and gases. Carbon monoxide and carbon dioxide are particularly hazardous, as they are colorless and odorless. Signs and symptoms vary with each type of exposure. Some cause eye irritation while others cause irritation of the respiratory tract. Move the victim into fresh air. If the victim is breathing without difficulty, call the Poison Control Center. If the victim is having trouble breathing or has other signs or symptoms of poisoning, call 911.

Absorbed Poisons

The three most common types of absorbed poisons are poison ivy, poison sumac, and poison oak. Exposure to any of these substances can cause itching, swelling, redness and blisters. Remove exposed clothing carefully and wash skin thoroughly with soap and water. Contact a physician for treatment.

If a chemical is spilled on the skin, remove exposed clothing and rinse the skin with warm water for at least 20 minutes. Contact the Poison Control Center.

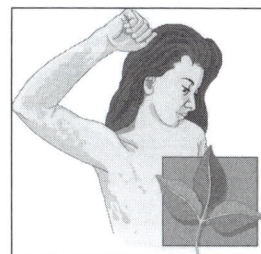

Substance Abuse

In 2001 there were 638,484 drug-related emergency department admissions in the US. Be aware that the signs and symptoms of poisoning may be due to substance abuse. Look for drug paraphernalia, empty pill or alcohol containers. Follow general poisoning treatment guidelines, and ensure escape route if patient becomes violent.

Confined Space Emergency

Confined spaces may contain an accumulation of flammable or toxic gases, many colorless and odorless. Hundreds of employees die each year in confined space accidents. Rescuers can become victims themselves because they need to get close to the victim in order to pull him or her out. Follow OSHA prescribed permit entry. Avoid becoming a victim; do not enter any confined space without proper equipment and training.

Heat-related emergencies are a true medical emergency. They occur most often in the early summer before people have become used to high temperatures. These emergencies commonly occur when the salt and water electrolyte balance in the body becomes skewed. Competitive athletes, laborers, alcoholics, obese people and soldiers are extremely susceptible to heat-related emergencies.

There are three types of heat emergency:

Heat Cramps – occur when a person sweats profusely and does not replace salt.

SIGNS AND SYMPTOMS:
- Hot, flushed skin
- Cramps in legs or abdomen

TREATMENT:
1. Remove from hot environment.
2. Gently stretch cramping muscles.
3. Massage cramps if indicated.
4. Replenish with water or sports drink.

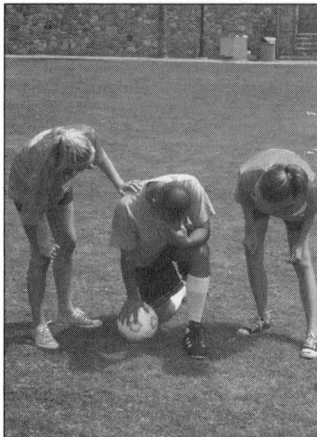

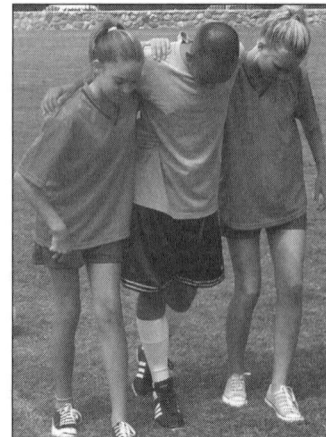

Heat Exhaustion – occurs when people work, exercise, or play in a hot, humid place. Body fluids are lost through sweating, causing the body to overheat.

SIGNS AND SYMPTOMS:
- Pale, clammy skin (sweating)
- Elevated temperature
- Intense thirst
- Fatigue and weakness
- Anxiety
- Headache
- Cramps

Heat Stroke – occurs when the body is unable to regulate its temperature. The body temperature rises rapidly and the cooling mechanism fails.

SIGNS AND SYMPTOMS:
- Body temperature above 104° F
- Hot, dry, flushed skin (may be sweating)
- Disoriented or unusual behavior
- Seizures
- Increased heart and respiratory rate
- Unresponsiveness

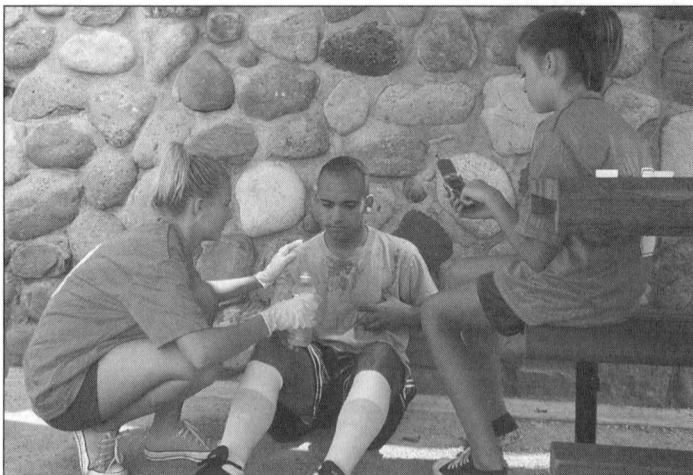

If the victim begins to shiver, slow the cooling efforts.

TREATMENT (HEAT EXHAUSTION/STROKE):
1. ABCD'S
2. Activate EMS (call 911).
3. Remove patient from hot environment.
4. Remove clothing.
5. Apply cooling measures (cool water, fan).
6. Monitor body temperature and condition.
7. Give water or sports drink if tolerated (no nausea, vomiting, seizure, or confusion).
8. DO NOT apply rubbing alcohol.
9. DO NOT give alcohol or caffeine drinks.
10. DO NOT give salt tablets.

HYPOTHERMIA

Immersion in cold water is the most common cause of hypothermia. It does not occur solely in extremely low temperatures. Cases have been recorded in temperatures as high as 65° F.

Death may result within hours of the first signs and symptoms. The greatest risk is to the elderly and very young, whose body temperature regulation mechanisms do not work as well or are not fully developed. Homeless people and those who are exposed to the elements are also at risk.

SIGNS AND SYMPTOMS:
- Shivering is the body's attempt to generate heat (will stop if the body core temperature drops below 90° F).
- Cold gray skin
- Drowsiness
- Slurred speech
- Exhaustion and unresponsiveness

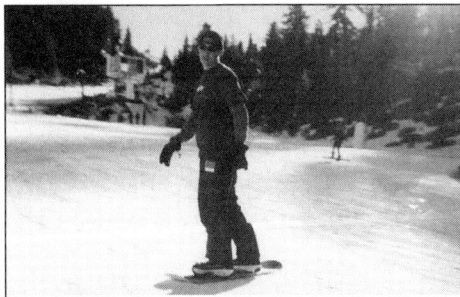

TREATMENT:
1. ABCD'S, activate EMS (call 911).
2. Remove from cold environment.
3. Remove damp clothing; replace with warm.
4. Insulate head – victim can lose up to 70% of body heat through the scalp.
5. Place victim in warm environment.
6. If far from medical care, warm with heat pads or containers of warm water. Keep a barrier between heat source and skin.
7. DO NOT manipulate extremities. Doing so forces cold blood back to the heart, which may result in cardiac arrest.
8. DO NOT give alcohol or coffee.

FROSTBITE

Frostbite is caused by prolonged exposure to cold as body tissues actually become frozen. As the tissue begins to freeze, ice crystals develop, damaging the cells in the frozen area. It most commonly affects the following areas:

- **Hands**
- **Feet**
- **Cheeks**
- **Ears**
- **Nose**

SIGNS AND SYMPTOMS:
- Pale, cold, waxy skin
- Painful, burning sensation, or numbness
- Blisters, hardened tissues

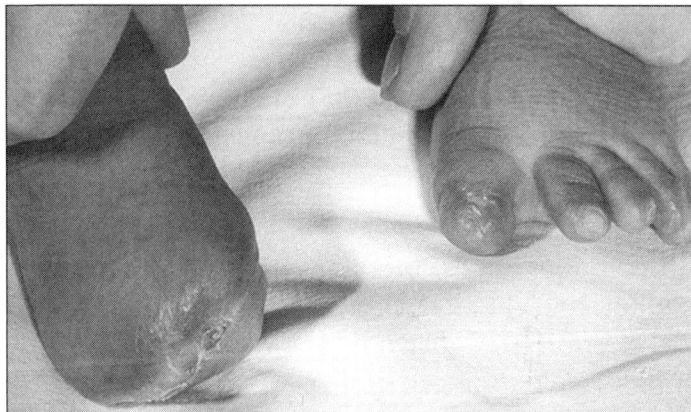

Results of frostbitten toes

TREATMENT:
1. ABCD'S
2. Activate EMS (call 911).
3. Remove victim from cold environment.
4. Remove wet clothing; replace with dry.
5. Place frostbitten part next to your body.
6. Remove rings, bracelets and watches.
7. Avoid partial thawing and refreezing.
8. DO NOT rewarm with a stove, open flame or heating pad.
9. DO NOT pop blisters.

ANIMAL BITES

Dogs are responsible for about 80% of all animal bites in the U.S. Most of the victims are younger than 10 years old. The primary concerns are bleeding and infection.

Rabies and tetanus are also a concern because there is no cure; immediate treatment is critical. A bite from a skunk, raccoon, bat, fox, or another mammal that is unprovoked or behaving strangely is treated as a rabies exposure.

Tips to avoid dog bites:

- If approached by a dog, stand still; do not run.
- Teach children not to annoy or tease animals.
- Be wary of moms with pups.
- Do not approach an unknown animal.
- Do not disturb an eating dog.
- Do not leave children or strangers alone with a dog.
- Do not attempt to break up a dog fight.

TREATMENT IF SKIN BROKEN:
1. Ensure scene safety. Do not touch or try to capture a potentially rabid animal.
2. Ask a bystander to call 911 and get a first aid kit.
3. Wash wound for several minutes with soap and water.
4. Control bleeding with direct pressure.
5. Apply triple antibiotic ointment and cover with a sterile dressing.
6. Seek medical care for further wound cleaning, sutures or vaccine.
7. Report bites to a police or animal control officer.

Human bites can occur during fights when skin on a knuckle is broken during a punch to the mouth, or when children are fighting or playing with each other. Human bites have the highest risk for infection.

SNAKEBITES

Snakebites can be painful, but most snakes are not poisonous. There are four types of poisonous snakes found in the U.S.: the rattlesnake, the coral snake, the cottonmouth (water moccasin), and the copperhead. Do not play with or pick up a snake unless you are properly trained. Consider all snakes as poisonous until proven otherwise. **Antivenin must be given within 4 hours of a bite.**

SIGNS AND SYMPTOMS:
- Fang marks (2 small puncture wounds)
- Burning pain
- Rapid swelling within minutes
- Nausea, vomiting
- Weakness
- Sweating

Poisonous snakes leave two puncture wounds.

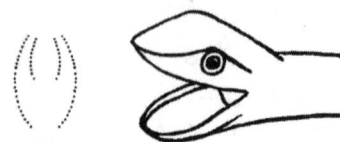

TREATMENT:
1. Consider scene safety.
2. Call 911 or local emergency number.
3. Keep the victim calm; decrease activity.
4. Wash the wound gently.
5. Immobilize the area, keeping it lower than the heart; remove jewelry.
6. For elapid snakebites (e.g. coral snake), wrap the entire limb snugly with a bandage, but loose enough for one finger to slip underneath.
7. Mark the border of the swelling/redness every 15 minutes with a pen.
8. DO NOT apply a tourniquet.
9. DO NOT cut wound or apply mouth suction or local electric shock.
10. DO NOT apply ice.

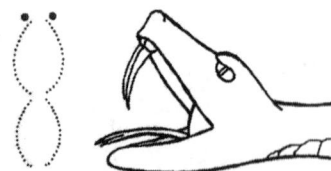

Nonpoisonous snakes leave a horseshoe shaped bite wound.

SPIDER BITES AND SCORPION STINGS

In the US, spider bites and scorpion stings are rare, and usually harmless to humans. Only two spiders (the brown recluse and the black widow) and one scorpion (the bark scorpion) pose a risk.

SIGNS AND SYMPTOMS:
- Severe pain, burning
- Swelling, rash, itching
- Small puncture wounds
- A blister or ulcer that may turn black
- Headache, dizziness, weakness
- Elevated heart rate and blood pressure
- Sweating, fever, cramps
- Nausea, vomiting, salivation
- Respiratory distress
- Anxiety, unresponsiveness

The Black Widow has a shiny black body with a red hourglass on its underside.

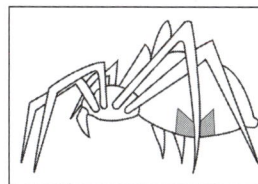

The Brown Recluse is light brown with a violin-shaped mark on its head and neck.

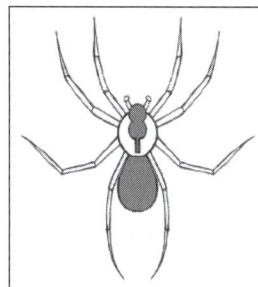

TREATMENT:
1. Follow the guidelines for snakebite.
2. Activate EMS.
3. Apply cold pack wrapped in a cloth.

TICK BITES

Ticks are related to spiders, and may carry serious diseases such as Lyme disease. Their bite is painless, so it is important to check your skin and clothing for them when coming indoors. Use repellant to prevent tick bites.

Tick Removal and Treatment:
- Remove as soon as possible.
- Use curved tweezers to grasp the tick close to the skin.
- Lift the tick straight out without twisting or pinching until it lets go.
- Save the tick for testing in a sealed container, if Lyme disease is prevalent in your area.
- Wash the site with soap and water and apply an antiseptic solution.
- Apply a cold pack.
- Seek medical care if you cannot remove the tick completely, or if a rash or flu-like symptoms develop.
- DO NOT use petroleum jelly, alcohol, or a hot match to kill the tick before removal.

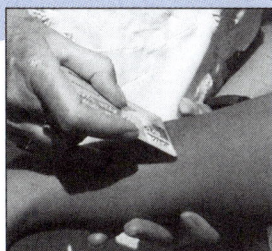

INSECT STINGS

Insect stings can cause pain, swelling, and allergic reactions. If a victim develops serious symptoms (breathing difficulties, severe swelling, hives, nausea or dizziness), seek medical help immediately.

If stung by a bee, quickly place your fingernail or a credit card at the base of the stinger and scrape it off.

Removing the stinger

You are at the lake and notice a woman who is having difficulty breathing. Her lips and face appear swollen. She states that she was stung by a bee, but already removed the stinger.

Place the action steps in correct sequence.

_____ Tell a bystander to call 911.

_____ Monitor ABCD'S for change in status.

_____ Help the patient use her epinephrine auto-injector, if requested and you are trained.

A coworker tells you that he splashed a strong chemical on his arm. He is not in distress or having trouble breathing.

Place the action steps in correct sequence.

_____ Rinse the skin with warm water for at least 20 minutes.

_____ Put on gloves and help the victim remove the contaminated clothing.

_____ Notify the company safety officer to obtain the MSDS.

_____ Contact the poison control center for further instructions.

_____ Monitor the ABCD'S. Activate EMS if the victim is in distress.

_____ Send a coworker to get the first aid kit.

Respond quickly to illness or injury – keep a first aid kit at home, in your vehicle and at work. Keep a current list of emergency phone numbers: police, fire, poison control, ambulance.

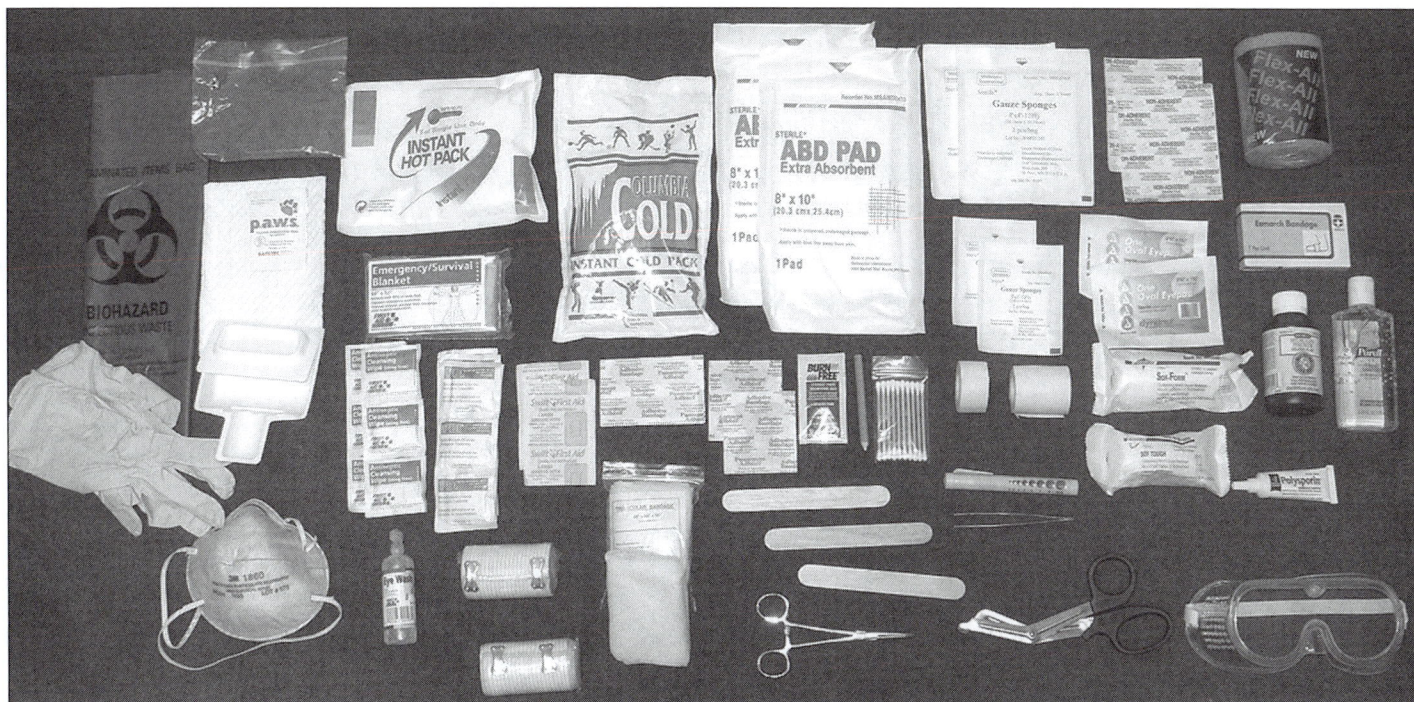

A Complete First Aid Kit Should Include:

- Personal Protective Equipment (PPE): disposable gloves, eye protection, CPR barrier devices, disposable gown, mouth/nose cover, anti-microbial wipes/gel

- Bleeding control: multi-size gauze pads, non-adherent dressings, multi-size roll gauze, tape, ABD pads, adhesive bandages of different sizes and types (i.e. finger, knuckle, butterfly)

- Injury Treatment: trauma shears, splint-roll, splinting supplies, cold pack, triangular bandages, elastic bandages

- Burn Care: burn sheet, burn gel, water, sterile dressings and gauze

- Bloodborne Pathogens Spill Kit: biohazard bag, rigid scoop/scraper, pick-up powder, disposable gloves, disposable apron, germicidal floor wipes

- Wound Care: tweezers, antibiotic ointment, antiseptic towellettes/cream, topical sting relief

- Miscellaneous: eyewash, sterile eye pads, tongue blades, hot pack, alcohol wipes, patient assessment form, first aid handbook

PREPARE BEFORE AN EMERGENCY OR DISASTER STRIKES!

FIRST AID KITS AND SUPPLIES

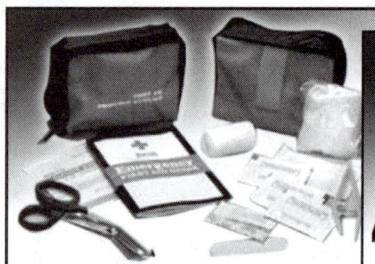

PERSONAL

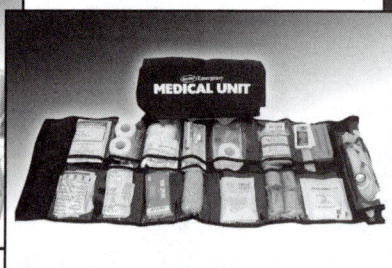

HOME

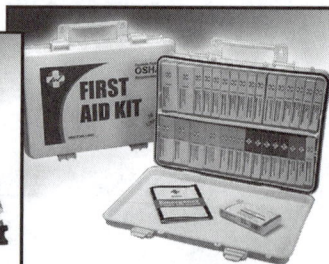

WORKPLACE

CPR BARRIER MASKS

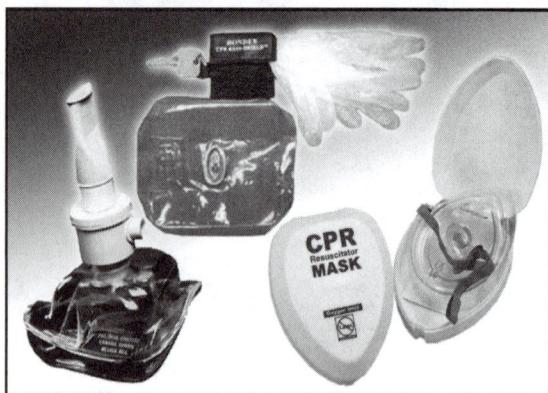

DISASTER READINESS

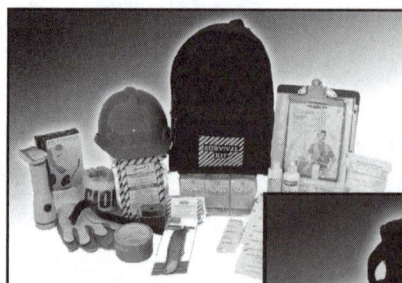

WORKPLACE

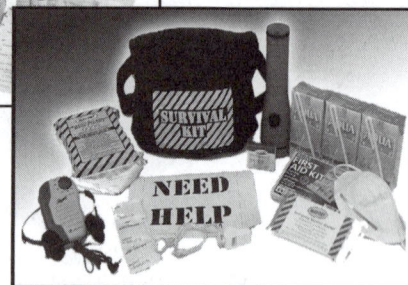

INDIVIDUAL

PET SAFETY

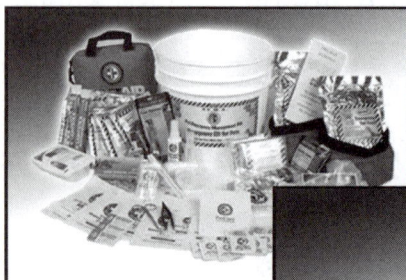

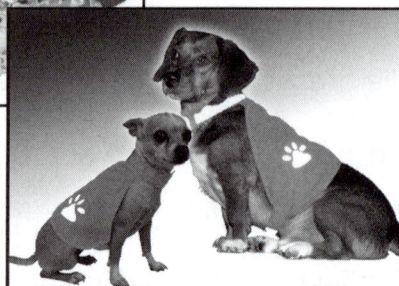

AED UNITS

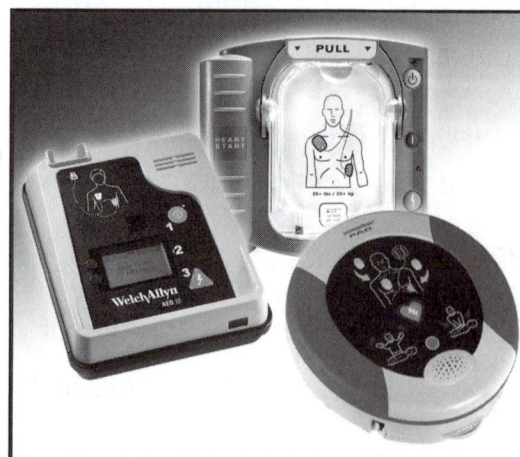

EMS SAFETY SERVICES
1-800-215-9555 www.emssafety.com

ORDER YOUR FIRST AID AND DISASTER READINESS PRODUCTS TODAY. CONTACT YOUR INSTRUCTOR OR VISIT WWW. EMSSAFETY.COM

AED/CPR Exam:

		T	F
1.	ABCD'S stand for Activate EMS, Breathing, Compressions, Defibrillation, and Severe allergic reaction.	☐	☑
2.	The depth of chest compressions on an adult is 1½ - 2 inches.	☑	☐
3.	The ratio of compressions to ventilations for all patients is 30:2.	☑	☐
4.	Lay rescuers should check for breathing during every cycle of CPR.	☐	☑
5.	After the AED delivers a shock, the rescuer should immediately resume CPR.	☑	☑
6.	Survival of cardiac arrest is more likely when effective CPR is combined with the early use of an AED.	☑	☐
7.	A rescuer should complete 5 cycles of CPR in about 2 minutes.	☑	☐
8.	Use the head tilt/chin lift maneuver to open the airway for all patients.	☑	☐
9.	Rescuers should spend 15 seconds looking, listening and feeling for breathing.	☑	☑
10.	A lay rescuer should check for a pulse before beginning chest compressions.	☐	☑
11.	If a choking victim is coughing forcefully, provide immediate abdominal thrusts.	☐	☑
12.	Clear a patient prior to pushing the shock button by making sure no one is touching the patient and loudly stating, "I'm clear. You're clear. We're all clear."	☑	☐
13.	The most important factor affecting a victim's survival is the presence of a trained rescuer who is equipped and willing to respond.	☑	☐
14.	If a patient starts to move after receiving a shock from an AED, remove the electrode pads and place in the recovery position.	☐	☑
15.	Never use pediatric electrode pads on an adult patient.	☑	☐

First Aid Exam:

		T	F
1.	The primary first aid treatment to control bleeding is direct pressure.	☑	☐
2.	Chemicals in the eyes should be flushed for at least 20 minutes.	☑	☐
3.	Always remove an impaled object to prevent further injury.	☐	☑
4.	The treatment for heat-related emergencies includes removing the victim from the environment and cooling him or her.	☑	☐
5.	Signs and symptoms of a heart attack include weakness on one side of the body, facial droop, confusion and slurred speech.	☐	☑
6.	Always place something in a seizure victim's mouth to prevent him or her from biting the tongue.	☐	☑
7.	DO NOT elevate the legs to treat for shock if you suspect a neck or back injury or a leg fracture.	☑	☐
8.	Straighten a fractured limb before applying a splint.	☐	☑
9.	The first priority in treating an unresponsive victim is to control bleeding.	☐	☑
10.	During an allergic reaction, the faster the onset of symptoms, the more severe the reaction.	☑	☐
11.	Cool a small or minor thermal burn with large amounts of cold water until pain decreases.	☑	☐
12.	If a victim has a head injury, assume there is also a neck injury.	☑	☐
13.	Induce vomiting after all exposures to ingested poisons.	☐	☑
14.	Remove the dressing over a bleeding wound frequently to see if bleeding has stopped.	☐	☑
15.	During an asthma attack, help the victim locate and use his or her inhaler.	☑	☐

EMS SAFETY SERVICES STUDENT AGREEMENT

1. I understand that emergency situations are inherently dangerous. I recognize the need to ensure my safety as well as that of the victim.   *Initial* ___

2. I understand the mode of transmission for bloodborne pathogens and recognize the need for gloves and CPR barrier devices. I have seen them demonstrated by a certified EMS Safety Services instructor.   *Initial* ___

3. I understand that if I come to the aid of an ill or injured person of my own free will, I am covered by the Good Samaritan Law.   *Initial* ___

4. I have practiced and feel comfortable with the skills and techniques taught in this EMS Safety Services training course.   *Initial* ___

My EMS Safety Services certified instructor was _Dee STueve_

FREDDy Sheehan   _(signature)_   _1/13/09_

Student Name (Print)   Student Signature   Date

SKILLS PERFORMANCE CHECKLIST

Instructor to initial each skill as student demonstrates proficiency.

AED/CPR:

___ ABCD'S

___ Recovery Position

___ Adult CPR

___ Child CPR*

___ Infant CPR*

___ AED Use

___ Adult/Child Choking

___ Infant Choking*

*Optional skill required for Pediatric certification.

First Aid:

___ Disposable Glove Removal

___ Patient Assessment for Illness or Injury

___ Control of Bleeding

___ Shock Position

___ Splinting Fractures